Inquiries should be addressed to:
Tom Robbins
Chapel Ministries Outreach
3054 W 400 N
Peru, IN 46970
www.chapelministriesoutreach.org

CONTENTS

A Tribute

I want to dedicate this book to my wife, Pam. She has faithfully stood beside me through all the ups and downs of ministry these past 23 years. She's been an exceptional wife and partner, an outstanding mother to our four sons Tom, Scott, Allen, and Kevin, a loving, caring mother-in-law to our daughters-in-law Trisha, Misty, and Abby, and a wonderful grandmother to our grandson Braxten and our granddaughter Addison.

I thank her with all my heart for her unwavering support during my five months of leukemia treatment. She provided amazing strength, comfort, and help during my most difficult times.

Proverbs 31:10 asks, "Who can find a virtuous woman?" And I can answer, "I have!"

Chapter One
A Little Background

I'm 51 years old and one of the few people fortunate enough to do something for a living my heart loves. I have been a pastor for 23 years, and I can honestly say that it is a vocation that I truly love with all of my heart. But if you seek to carry the burdens of others, to shepherd, lead, and help others through all the problems of life, you'll find it to be a stressful job that takes its toll. I've experienced this in my own life and some of what I have experienced is a result of my own lack of obedience to Philippians 4:6:

> *Be anxious for nothing, but in everything by prayer and supplication, with thanksgiving, let your requests be made known to God . . .*

I was born into the home of a very godly family. My father, Jack Robbins, and my mother, Virginia Robbins, were known in the community to be one of the most godly couples around.

My father had a prophet's anointing. He had a special presence about him. I enjoyed being with him even though, as a young child, I didn't spend a lot of time with him. He was busy. He, like many fathers, later regretted not being able to spend as much time with his children as he should—an easy pitfall for a minister.

Dad was a man of integrity, a man who cared about people. He was gifted with wisdom. I know of people who drove three or four hours just to ask for a half-hour's worth of advice. Daddy was a tremendous preacher with great insight into God's Word. He was a man of prayer. He was also a manic-depressive beset

1

with a lot of emotional trauma. During his ministry, he had two nervous breakdowns. But, in spite of that weakness, God used him in tremendous ways. I often think of my father (and myself) when I read II Corinthians 12:9:

My strength is made perfect in weakness.

We were trained by our mother. I look back and realize the value of a godly mother. Just over five feet tall, all German, and a powerhouse of a woman, she was one to protect and care for her children! But, most of all, she wanted them to have a godly foundation.

During the early years of my life, my father was a traveling evangelist. I distinctly remember him being gone, ministering somewhere in the Midwest night after night. I have vivid memories of my mother going to her room to pray for him every evening about 7:00 or 7:30 (when Daddy would be beginning his revival services). Then she would invite us into her room and tell us Bible stories. An animated person with an outgoing personality, she was a superb storyteller. I can't begin to tell you the long-term importance of hearing the stories of David and Goliath, of Daniel in the lion's den, and of Jesus and His disciples. As she took us through the Bible, she not only told us the stories, but acted them out in a way that made an indelible impression on our young minds. She had us memorizing Scripture before we could barely talk. At two or three years of age we knew Scripture verses by heart.

There is no way of calculating the value of such a spiritual foundation. As a grown man who's observed lots of families, I can't begin to measure the value of a mother who teaches her children the "ways of the Lord."

Many people take the view that only a preacher or Sunday School teacher can teach Bible stories. They underestimate the incredible impact a child experiences when they hear the stories from their parent. It impacted me. And at an early age, I felt God tugging at my heart. The Scripture had definitely taken root, prompting me to go to the altar at Daddy's revival meetings many times because of God's tug.

During the summer months we traveled with Dad and participated musically in his revival meetings. I'm amused at some of the things we did. Daddy didn't make much money. To save fuel, he drove a Volkswagen beetle that pulled a small trailer. Though I have six siblings, only three of us were still at home. Carroll, Miriam, and I sat in the backseat, with me in the middle, while Dad and Mom sat up front. We traveled all over the United States. I still don't believe we traveled in such small quarters, but we did!

I remember the long hours, as Daddy would finish a meeting in Pennsylvania then drive us to Nebraska for a meeting that started a day and a half later. Mom would sing to pass the time. We each would sing. We all learned to sing each other's harmony parts because of the hours we traveled together. And those experiences bonded us into a close family unit. My heart goes out to children who are raised on TV and video games. They don't experience the joy that comes from really knowing and loving others.

I must tell you of a unique experience I had at eight years of age. Daddy was "on the road," so Mom took us to a little church in Majenica, Indiana, a Christian and Missionary Alliance Church. A missionary who ministered in Baliem Valley, New Guinea, showed us pictures of indigenous people—primitive and very poor people—who had never heard the Gospel. And I was startled by the fact that none of them wore clothes! But, something powerful happened to me. As he showed pictures of poor, unkempt, and unclothed children, my heart was deeply touched. I remember going home in tears. I cried and cried and cried. My mother became quite concerned because several days went by and I was still going off by myself and having crying spells. She was intuitive enough to realize that something spiritually significant was taking place—that God was tugging on my heart about the needs of people.

Although I thought I was going to be a missionary, it was not what God was calling me to do. Rather, he was stirring my heart about the needs of people. And that stirring continued to grow. After that experience I remember practicing preaching and visualizing myself as a missionary or pastor. It became my goal.

Unfortunately, I strayed from my calling during the teenage years and became angry and bitter over some of the difficult circumstances of life. A number of things contributed to my prodigal years, including the sudden, unexpected death of my sister Carroll. A couple of years after marrying and having her first child, she went to the doctor for a simple surgical procedure, suffered a massive reaction to the anesthetic (it happens to one in ten thousand people) and died on the operating table. To this day I can't put into words how much Carroll meant to me, and how devastating it was to lose her.

There are other stories I could tell, but suffice it to say, I returned to the Lord at 18 years of age, just before my 19th birthday. God heard the prayers of my family, especially my mother, and drew me back to himself. I'm so grateful for God's patience with me. The deep desire to be the best Christian I could ever be, the desire he placed in my heart as a child, remained intact and intense. And the call to minister to hurting people was still alive.

I remember sitting in church observing people who professed to be Christians, but didn't seem to be fully engaged with the Lord. Though they wore the label of a disciple, they didn't seem to want to be a disciple. I decided if I was going to be a Christian, I wanted to be the best I could be. I wanted to "go for the gold" and grow as close to the Lord as I could in true discipleship. I'm thankful for that desire. I'm not sure where that desire originated; God just put it in me. This God-placed desire saw me through a nervous breakdown in my early 20's. Even though I could hold down a job and do the normal day-by-day things of life, I struggled with emotional problems to the point that I would experience uncontrollable crying spells almost daily. In this difficult time I began to develop a stronger bond with the Lord through the study of his word and prayer.

In Psalms 51 it says, "God is nigh unto them of a broken spirit." I was broken. And through prayer, God was near. This reality cannot be over emphasized. Prayer was my strength. Developing a prayer life was foundational for me.

With the family raised, my father and mother felt called to missionary work and left for Haiti. I admire them greatly for being willing to tackle the difficulties of a third-world country at their age. Meanwhile, Pam and I tackled parenting. At 22 years of age, we already had two sons, Tom and Scott.

Still needing mentoring, God crossed my path with a very godly man by the name of Ronald Bishop. Pastor Bishop (my name for him) had ministered in British Honduras were he buried two of his sons. His wife suffered severe neurological trauma but remained alive in a comatose state for six years. Her condition required him to return to the United States where he pastored a church in Fort Wayne, Indiana. This godly man, one so determined to stay true to the Lord and his calling, intrigued me. Though pastoring a church, and still raising three daughters, Pastor Bishop would visit his wife daily, and with hymnal in hand he would sing to her. He faithfully cared for her until she died, and then moved to my community, Peru, Indiana, to pastor a church.

Sensing that God was dealing with me about vocational ministry, I began attending the church he pastored, and an incredible, God-ordered friendship began to blossom—we really connected! I think his desire for a son and my need for a father and mentor were the perfect match.

God orders things in our lives. It's no coincidence that he became my mentor. Here I was, working third shift in the local Kroger store, starting a young family, wondering how things would develop in my life, and wondering what way I should go when Pastor Bishop took me under his wing!

His mentoring started with prayer. It was his practice to have devotions at his church early in the morning. Since I worked third shift, I began meeting with him every morning and having prayer with him. We would sit on the floor near the altar and talk, or cry, or pray. There's no simple way to express the value of those times as I saw him cry and pray. Pastor Bishop had a better understanding of compassion—the compassion of Christ—than anyone I've ever met.

The Bible says we learn obedience through the things we suffer. I think his suffering caused him to develop this marvelous compassion. The Bible also says we are not to waste our sorrows, and I believe Pastor Bishop's sorrows—the deaths of his sons, the long illness and death of his wife—refined him into pure gold!

Romans 8:28 tells us, *"For we know in all things God works for good . . ."*

I was both intrigued and challenged by this man. Though there was a deep desire within me to be a world-class Christian and practice a strong prayer life, this desire needed to be mentored. It required someone of tremendous faith and stability, a man who knew suffering but maintained a tender, Christ-like spirit. Pastor Bishop was that someone, a mentor whose entire life was about relationships—his relationship with God and his relationship with others.

We spent two years together and I helped in his church. Then God called him to a pastorate in Ohio. It was difficult for me to see him go, but I look back now and realize it was time for me to stand on my own two feet.

Shortly after he left (by then I was 24 years old with 3 children), God led me to pastor a small, local church on a part-time basis for one year. Until that time, I had been doing some guest speaking and was leading various Bible studies. Though I was not ready for pastoral leadership, it was great experience. My wife and I led singing and taught bible classes, I preached every Sunday, while continuing to work part-time at the local Kroger store.

Following that year of pastoral ministry, I went back to fulltime work at Kroger for the next four years. I experienced a lot of frustration wondering why ministry opportunities weren't opening up for me. Instead, I found myself promoted to a supervisory position and spent a lot of stressful hours working at a very demanding job. Looking back, I realize God was putting me through a "seminary" of his own choosing. He was preparing me for the demanding task of leading and shepherding people.

It wasn't until I was 29 years of age that my desire to minister fulltime became reality. An opportunity developed for me to pastor another small, local church. And our fourth son, Kevin, was born.

So, we were a young couple with four children, with no formal ministerial training, stepping into full time pastoral ministry. All I can say is that God was clearly leading us and he confirmed his leading with his blessing. In two short years our church grew from 25 to 150 people. We had to relocate to a new building, and were accepted into a major denomination. This was a Godsend for it enabled me to get some much needed schooling, as well as ordination credentials.

In the following years, our church became a unique ministry. I'm not sure of all the reasons God puts certain things on one's heart, but I've always felt I was to minister to anyone of any kind and in any condition. I found myself especially sensitive and drawn to those who were down and out and needed another chance.

In the Gospels, Jesus speaks about a great feast that was prepared by a generous overlord. Many were invited, but they made a multitude of excuses and wouldn't come. So he sent his servants out to bring in the maimed, the halt, and the blind, because, "my table will be full." Even after they had combed the community, the servants came to the lord and said there was room for more. He responded, "You go out into the highways and hedges and you compel them. You make them come in. Bring in the highways and hedges people, the people who are troubled. My table will be filled."

That passage of Scripture resonates with me. I've always felt it is what my ministry is supposed to be. And that is what our church became. A nurse in our congregation accurately described us by saying if all the churches in the community were to combine and become a hospital, our church would be the emergency room! That's what it was. We ministered to a lot of helpless, hurting, and bleeding people.

It was a stressful pastorate, as "emergency room" type ministry always is. It's filled by people with lots of problems—addictions, broken marriages, broken families, broken lives. But, I felt this was something I was supposed to do. This was my calling, my kind of people. Ten years later, the church had grown to 400 people. We had to use a video screen for the people seated in an overflow room.

8

During this same ten-year period, an incredible series of things happened that became tremendous heartaches for my wife and me. Our second son rebelled against the way he was raised. A lot like a teenaged me, he decided that he had to make his own way. Deeply hurt through a variety of high school experiences, he developed a bitterness toward God and fell away from Him. Because he had developed a bad reputation in our community and needed a fresh start, I suggested that he go Seattle, Washington, where my sister Sharon and her husband Steve lived. Steve was a youth minister of a large church and was willing to look after him. So, when he turned 18 and graduated from high school, he took me up on my suggestion and moved west.

The plan didn't work. Our son became even more wayward, moved out of my sister's home and began living on the streets. He became a drug addict—a main-line cocaine and heroin user. At one point, we heard he had been rescued by a "street girl" when he overdosed. It was heartbreaking. We were in the valley of despair. I can remember my wife crying night after night. I ended up going to Seattle and combing the streets for him.

During this tough time, and to complicate matters, our third son was severely injured in an automobile accident while leaving the local high school. With multiple brain injuries, he was airlifted by helicopter to Methodist Hospital in Indianapolis where he remained near death for days. I'll never forget the exact words the neurosurgeon used: "He has more hemorrhages on his brain than we can count. The best you can expect—if he lives, and I don't think he will—is that he will be totally paralyzed on one side." We lived at the hospital for weeks. It was a difficult time compounded by financial stress. But God cared for us in a tremendous way. It's amazing how God looks after his own. In the Psalms we read, "Many are the afflictions of the righteous, but the Lord delivers him out of them all."

9

Our son was in a coma for quite a period of time and it was difficult to tell how he was doing. I remember going to his room the second night praying that he would live and not be paralyzed. Standing alone in the intensive care unit, with tears running down my face, I prayed, "Lord, would you give me some idea of how this is going to go. Could you just give me some sign?"

Out of the corner of my eye I saw him move his toe on the side of his body the doctor thought would be permanently paralyzed. Being a doubting Thomas, as I often am, I thought I had imagined what I saw. I prayed, "Lord, if that's really what happened, cause it to happen again." It happened again. I called to the nurse who was on the other side of the glass window and told her our son had moved. She said, "He did?" I said, "Yes." She said, "Maybe it's just a reflex." And as she began to rub the calf of his leg, he kicked at her, a deliberate action. And I joyfully lapsed into one of the hardest crying spells I'd had for a long time, realizing that he wasn't paralyzed.

In addition to large miracles, numerous smaller miracles occurred. We had asked the Lord for financial help because medical care of the kind we needed was expensive. The first three days, relatives and friends from the church began visiting us. Often they would stick some cash in my pocket and say, "Here, use this however." On the third day, I began counting the cash to see how much had been given. It totaled $5,400. I was stunned. God had started to provide for the three months we would be at the hospital—Jehovah Jireh, the provider, the one who sees ahead.

Since the doctor told us Allen might not live, we decided to ask our sons to come home. Our oldest son, Tom, was in college in Minnesota; Scott was somewhere in the Seattle area—we weren't sure where; Kevin, our youngest son, was still at home. We sent someone looking for Scott. When he stepped off the hospital elevator, I knew immediately he was a drug addict. He could not have weighed more than 85 pounds.

Again, Romans 8:28 tells us that God works all things for good: "For we know that in all things God works for the good of those who love him and are called according to His purpose." It was through Allen's accident that Scott came home. It was through that difficult series of events that Scott went into rehabilitation for 13 months, and is now serving the Lord and doing well. Allen, our walking medical miracle, is totally recovered. He graduated from college in 2005, is married and working in a church in Oklahoma! Pam and I remain so grateful for God's faithfulness.

The church continued to grow and I started to feel overwhelmed with the army of new Christians that had joined our ranks. I needed more staff help to accomplish all that needed to be done. It was during this time that God began speaking to me about greater involvement with the "down and out." Through a video produced by our denomination, I felt moved to minister to inner-city people. I was drawn to visit inner city Chicago and began to feel that God was leading me to leave my church and move to Chicago. It was a leading fraught with family complications and vocational uncertainties. In some ways, it seemed to defy common sense. Leaving my church in central Indiana and moving to the concrete jungle of Chicago were two of the hardest things I would ever do.

Though many friends didn't fully understand this leading, we ministered for two years to the "outcasts" of society, working the streets at night from 11:00 p.m. until 3:00 a.m. We ministered to the homeless, prostitutes, and runaway kids. We converted a storefront building into a coffee house and held services for the "down and out" every Friday night.

It was during this time that I had another nervous breakdown. I had let the stress of pastoring an understaffed growing church build to an emotional breaking point. In retrospect, I believe it's why God led me to Chicago and gave me lots of help from Moody Bible Institute students who wanted to be trained in street ministry. My passion was still in full force—ministering to hurting people—but, rather than looking after 400 people, I was ministering one-on-one while giving guidance to these wonderful, dedicated students. The responsibility was one tenth of what it had been, and it gave me a chance to be alone, fall apart, cry through a few things, and spend more time in prayer.

Once again, God worked all things for good. While it was difficult to leave the church we loved, God knew I needed a break, a halftime in my life that wouldn't divert me from my calling of ministering to hurting people.

Sensing I needed a complete ministry break, I decided to take a six-month sabbatical. This seemed possible as I saw how effectively God was using others to lead our street ministry. Not knowing how I would handle a six-month sabbatical financially, I went to prayer. The very day that I promised God that I would take six months off, not having any idea how I would pay my bills, friends of ours called and invited us to their home. After a bit of friendly chitchat, they told me that they felt I needed a break, that I needed to get some rest, and that they wanted to give me $25,000 on one condition—I couldn't do anything for six months. I had to rest. I'll never forget the euphoric feeling I had knowing that Jehovah Jireh, the God who provides, who sees ahead, was providing for me. What an incredible privilege and blessing!

During those six months, I was able to put myself back together, spending hours in prayer. God helped me double my prayer time and I grew to know the Lord in new and wonderful ways.

As the six months came to an end, a longing began to develop to pastor again. While praying about these feelings, my elderly father (who was temporarily pastoring a small, rural church of about 25 people near Peru, Indiana) called me and asked if I would come and speak on Easter Sunday.

I was excited about this opportunity since I hadn't done much speaking for several months. On Resurrection Sunday Pam and I arrived at Skinner Chapel, a little country church started in the 1800's by a family named Skinner. The small sanctuary was full, and I will always remember the way I felt; I felt more at home than I had felt in years. While on the platform, I had the feeling I was in my living room. Even though I had never been to this church before, I knew this feeling of familiarity was something from God. He was leading me into a new chapter of ministry. Ministering here was something I was supposed to do. And through a sequence of events, much prayer, and the prompting of a couple of godly men in the church, I was invited to become the pastor. I'll always be grateful to Herbert Tomson and Paul Troyer.

Since my elderly father was experiencing some health problems, he fully affirmed that I should take his place. So, I became the pastor and have been there for the past eight years. The church has grown from 25-30 people to nearly 300. We have built two buildings in addition to the original sanctuary. We are a unique, rural ministry—a country church "emergency room." And we thank God for his blessing upon us. But it's not about us; it's about being obedient to God's plan for us.

13

Chapter 2

Who Goes Deer Hunting When They're Sick?

It was the first week of November 2005, and I was exhausted. For several months I had been showing signs of accumulating fatigue. My signs of tiredness prompted some of our church leaders to kid with me about getting older. I had turned 50 that year and often made light of my tiredness by blaming it on hitting the half-century mark. Though I didn't say so, I felt the personal counseling load I was carrying—many of these counseling situations were quite stressful—exacerbated the tiredness of my fifty year-old mind and body. I had no idea I was dealing with the growing symptoms of a major disease.

Often I would drive the 60 miles to Warren, Indiana, to visit my father, a resident of the Methodist home for the elderly. I was mystified by the need to take a half-hour nap in the waiting room in order to have the strength to drive home and finish out the day.

During the second week of November, my fatigue seemed more intense and I was experiencing some dizziness. A flu bug was going around that caused many people to feel weak, dizzy, and lightheaded. I concluded that, in addition to my "normal" fatigue, I had picked up this strain of flu. I became quite sick and had to cancel a number of visitations and counseling appointments. I stayed home from mid-week services Wednesday evening and rested all day Thursday. Nevertheless, I developed a migraine headache that lasted 22 hours. It wasn't until the headache dissipated that I found some relief, though I remained exhausted.

November 12 was opening day of shotgun deer season. I have

always loved hunting. I had begun deer hunting eight years before, taught by a couple of men in the church I was instrumental in leading to the Lord. My motive for hunting with them, in addition to my love for hunting itself, was to spend time with them and enrich our friendship.

But there was a third reason. I believe Christians can find tremendous guidance, comfort, and strength through their passions, as long as God is first in their lives and other things don't crowd Him out. I have had God speak to me in remarkable ways—through church services, through my prayer walks, and through people who mentored and encouraged me. Some of my very best times with God have been while deer hunting, especially during bow season.

For me there's nothing quite as soothing or relaxing to the spirit as slipping through a cornfield into a woods, hiding 20 feet off the ground in a deer stand, while watching the sun sink beneath the western horizon. God has given me direction many, many times in such a setting. My mother seemed to understand this side of me better than anyone. As my very best friend, she seemed to grasp my passion for hunting, my enjoyment of riding motorcycles, and encouraged me to do so—activities many mothers might not encourage, especially the love for motorcycles! Mom seemed to know the kind of heart I have and the kind of respite I needed. I have very fond memories of the special things she did for me, particularly with regard to hunting season.

Here's a very graphic example. During the years Pam and I ministered in Chicago, I came back to central Indiana for a week of deer hunting as a way to escape the burdens and stress of the streets and our kind of inner-city ministry. This one particular year, the opening morning of shotgun season was spectacular. It was about 30 degrees, and a wet snow had begun to fall just about daybreak.

15

I was hunting, with permission, on the farm of our dear friends, Orville and Helen Garber. Their woods were like a paradise—pure white snow sticking to the tree limbs in very unusual ways. When the sky cleared, and the sun came out, it was like sitting in a breathtaking stained glass window sanctuary. About 8:00 a.m., with binoculars in hand, I saw two does about 200 yards away, with a buck chasing after them. After some 30 minutes of staying close together, the buck, as though someone had kicked him, jumped up and started to run right toward me. When he came to the fence, he jumped it and stood statuesquely just 30 yards away. Though deer can do unusual things, I thought his behavior was most unusual. Seizing the moment, I slowly and calmly raised my shotgun and fired. He was, indeed, the nicest buck I had taken up to that time.

After dressing the deer and heading for home, I stopped as I often did to show the deer to my mother. She came out of the front door all excited, wanting to see the deer, cheering for me, smiling, and saying how glad she was that I had been successful.

Then she asked me an unusual question: "What time was it when you shot the deer?" I told her it had been right after 8:00a.m. She said that at that time, she had been in her room praying, "Heavenly Father, it makes me happy when my children are happy. I'm delighted when my children do well and achieve success. Please give Tom success in hunting this morning. He's been working hard in the ministry. Now he's come back here to relax. Please give him success this morning."

I asked Mom, "What time did you say you were you praying?"

She said, "It would have been around 8:00 a.m."

I said, "Mom, that's when the buck turned and ran toward me!"

My mother passed away at Christmastime five years ago from influenza complications. Realizing she was very sick, she uncharacteristically called me at 2:30 in the morning and asked me to come to her home, some seven miles away. I hopped out of bed, revved up my automobile, and discovered I was in a midst of a heavy, blinding snowstorm. The drifts were so bad that I got stuck on the road to her house and ended up walking to her door. I found her sitting on the couch, extremely congested, gasping for air. She asked me to help her to the bathroom. I faced her, put my arms around her, pulled her to me, and started walking backwards, pulling her down the hall to the bathroom.

How good God is in situations like these. At the time I didn't realize that those four or five minutes it took me to slowly walk her to the bathroom was God's way of allowing me to give her a five-minute hug, because it was destined to be the last one.

After she came back from the bathroom, I led her to a chair in the back bedroom, picked up the phone, and called a good friend to bring his four-wheel drive truck so we could take Mom to the hospital. Road conditions were too bad for an ambulance. While on the phone to him, I saw her struggling frantically, and realized that she had aspirated stomach fluids into her windpipe and was fatally choking. I tried my best to help her, but was unsuccessful. She died in my arms.

I laid her body back into a chair and sat down on the floor beside her. I'll never forget the hour and a half as I waited for the highway department to clear the road so a funeral director could come and take her body. I spent most of that time thanking God for such a godly mother. I also spent some time wondering why this had happened, and why I was unsuccessful in saving her life. But those questions don't haunt me, for, while sitting on the floor next to her, God spoke to me so plainly that I have never questioned what happened. He whispered to me, "Tom, as precious a Christian as your mother is, do you think that anything you did or didn't do would have changed what I wanted to do?" I realized then and there, with great emotion, that Mom was the property of the Lord, and that he had chosen to take her.

17

The following week I shared the funeral with my older brothers Paul and Jim, both ministers, and sang with my sisters Sharon and Miriam. What a privilege it was for the four of us to sing together and celebrate the life, ministry, and legacy of our dear mother. We all still miss her. Daddy, with his health rapidly deteriorating, missed her most of all.

The following autumn I went hunting once again on Garber's farm. Late one evening, sitting in the same exact tree stand I had been in the morning that Mom prayed, I began reflecting on a summer and early fall that had been especially difficult. Some serious tensions and difficult struggles related to our ministry had made for a difficult year. For several months I had found myself asking, "Why am I having such a hard time? Is it because Mom is gone? Mom always prayed for me and she's no longer here. Is that what is wrong?"

On a lesser note, this deer-hunting season had been one of my worst. I had hunted through the entire bow season with no success. My passion had turned to pain and frustration. Standing in the tree stand, I said to myself, "Well, my hunting success is probably over. Mom isn't here to pray for me."

About 30 seconds later, right at twilight, I heard a noise. I stood as still and breathless as possible. A beautiful eight-point buck came through the thicket about five feet from my tree and stood directly in front of me. I slowly turned, fired, and got the deer. The moment the buck fell, the Lord whispered and said, "Your Mom is gone, but I am not." I just broke down and had a glorious crying spell in the tree stand. No one will ever know what it meant to me to hear God faithfully affirm that, though Mom wasn't present, he was!

As you can see from these stories, my mother played an incredible role in my life by affirming my passions, often the means God has used to communicate with me. I don't feel

Christians are to ever feel guilty about things they enjoy—golfing, fishing, gardening, workouts, or a multitude of other activities—if those things are kept in their proper place. As long as we follow Matthew 6:33 and *"Seek first the kingdom of God and his righteousness,"* we can expect *"all things will be added to you."* My experience has taught me that God often uses the activities and experiences we love as a means of speaking to us in powerful ways. It will be on the golf course that a life-changing lesson will be taught, or at the fishing hole that an awesome prayer moment will occur. God meets us where we are and uses the normal, everyday moments of life to guide and direct us.

Perhaps all of the above might help explain why, though I was feeling very sick the second week of November 2005, I still had such an intense desire to go hunting on the opening day of deer season. Feeling quite weak, I compromised, and instead of hunting on Garber's farm, I decided to hunt directly behind my house. Choosing a deer stand about 100 yards behind my barn, I climbed up into it.

Once again, it was a spectacular, sunlit morning. Facing east, I saw eleven deer too far away for a shot. It didn't matter, for I just spent the time talking with God. But growing weary from standing, I sat down in the stand. Around 10:00 a.m. the most amazing thing happened, the significance of which I didn't grasp at the time or fully understand until much later.

As I was sitting and enjoying the morning, a breeze began to blow just loud enough to penetrate the silence. When hunting, you depend a lot on silence and your ability to hear an approaching deer. Suddenly, out of nowhere, a voice (not an impression, but an actual, audible voice) said, "Get up and turn around." It startled me. Obediently, without questioning the voice or giving it deliberative thought, I very, very slowly began to turn, raising myself on one knee, and stretching to stand. As I stood and looked over the limb behind me, I saw a beautiful buck

19

standing in the field behind me. I raised my gun and fired. The deer ran ten or twelve yards and fell into the creek. I climbed down from the stand, crossed the fence, and went to the deer, feeling increasingly faint. But in an instant, everything became very bright as though my eyes were dilated. The sky was blinding and the green grass looked yellow. Turning to walk away from the deer and head for the house, I collapsed on the ground. My first thought was that I was having a stroke. I didn't know what to do but lie there while asking God to help me get back to the house. After several minutes I got up and stumbled my way to the house, stopping several times to rest. It was in those moments that I first realized there might be something seriously wrong with me.

I approached the house thinking about hearing an audible voice and experiencing a collapse. As I went in, my wife greeted me, said she had heard the shotgun discharge, and asked if I had gotten a deer. Her question took me directly to the audible voice in the tree stand, flooded my heart with emotion, and I began to cry. She wanted to know what was wrong. I told her I had experienced something awesome and tried to explain how deeply my heart had been touched because God had audibly spoken to me in a tree stand. I was overwhelmed that the God of the universe would be interested enough in my wellbeing and everyday life to speak to me about a deer by telling me to stand up and turn around. I also told her I had collapsed in the field, but I wasn't crying about falling, I was crying because of the unfathomable privilege of hearing God speak to me audibly.

I decided to wait a couple of hours until my son could come and retrieve the deer, for I was too weak to do it myself. Instead, I went to bed for the rest of the day. A good friend who always helps me, Guy Woodhouse, the man who taught me to hunt, came to the house and took care of the deer for me.

I got up the next morning, Sunday, November 13 with the

intention of going to church and leading the service. But I had to call my assistant pastor, Chris Edgington, to lead the service in my place because I was too weak to go to church. I stayed in bed all day. Chris called to say that a sister of a good friend in our church had gotten very sick and was in a coma at Parkview Hospital in Fort Wayne. I knew Stephanie Van Baalen's concern for her sister Carmen would be very great, so I prayed through the night for Carmen.

Monday morning, feeling a little better, I drove to Fort Wayne. By the time I arrived at the hospital, some 60 miles away, I remember needing to rest in the parking garage before going inside. I found my way to the intensive care unit and anointed and prayed for Carmen. She died later in the week. Nevertheless, I believe God wanted me to anoint and pray for her. I have found that God sometimes calls us to minister when we do not feel capable to do so. Jesus set the example by ministering though weary to the bone. Tuesday morning I felt much better, so I drove to Kokomo to visit Helen Garber (the woman who owns the woods I hunt in). She was seeing her oncologist, Doctor Becker, at Howard Community Hospital Cancer Center. I spent an hour and a half with Helen and Orville. This meeting was also meant to be. God was preparing me for the days ahead. As you will see in the next chapter, Jehovah Jireh plans and prepares us for the future.

Jehovah Jireh is an Old Testament name that means, the "God who provides." The word provide comes from the root word _vid_. This is the root from which we derive the words visual and video. It means to see. I believe the true meaning of Jehovah Jireh is "the God who sees ahead." Looking back, I know there were so many instances where God was preparing me for what was coming. The list is a long one. Sitting for an hour and half in the Cancer Center with Helen Garber was definitely part of that preparation.

21

Another way "the God who sees ahead" was preparing me for what was coming involved prayer partners. I've always felt prayer partners were invaluable. I encourage people in our church to find a prayer partner—someone with whom you can share your thoughts, someone you can call on, someone devoted and committed to praying for you, your family, and your needs. These partnerships are invaluable to Christian living. We all need the encouragement and support of others. I find it interesting that when Jesus commissioned his followers, he sent them out as twos. A quotation I saw years ago says, "A friend doubles our joys and divides our grief." How true! We need the encouragement of other people. *"As iron sharpens iron, so one man sharpeneth another."* [Proverbs 27:17]

I felt compelled to enlist several prayer partners. Bryan Jaberg had been an accountability and prayer partner for several years; Matt Hunt, a quadriplegic and dear friend who has suffered greatly; and my brother-in-law Dave Hinds. Dave came to me and said God wanted him to do more in the area of prayer and asked if he could pray for me? I felt I should enroll him as a prayer partner. Dave calls me every Wednesday to remind me that Wednesday is his day to pray for me all day. What a contribution to ministry!

It is no coincidence that, in the year I found I had contracted acute myeloid leukemia (AML), was facing death, and might leave this world rather quickly, I would feel a strong need for prayer partners. Jehovah Jireh sees ahead. He knows what we need ahead of time. This was a year when I would need extra prayer.

It's important for the reader to know that I believe there was much more to AML than my physical peril. ***I believe with all my heart that my acute myeloid leukemia was an attack on the ministry.*** In the New Testament book of Ephesians it says, *"We fight not against flesh and blood but against principalities and* powers." Our spiritual enemy, Satan, is committed to destroying us in any way he can. I have always been humbled by realizing that God entrusted me with his truth—preaching the truth from the pulpit and sharing the truth with people through counseling. Satan is the antithesis of truth. Jesus said he is the father of all lies. Because Satan is committed to destroying truth, spiritual warfare requires much prayer. The God who sees ahead prompted me to seek out prayer partners.

It's also interesting how God used music to prepare me for what was coming. Music was bred into me and my brothers and sisters. There's no way to measure how much music has added to my life. During the months of September and October 2005, I had songs flowing through my memory nonstop. Many of us have had a song cycle endlessly through our mind to the place where it is annoying. This was different. These were songs that made their way through my head, to my heart, and to my soul!

One of those songs is *Rescue*. The lyrics read, "I need you, Jesus, to come to my rescue. Where else can I go? There's no other name by which I am saved. Capture me with grace." The words to *Rescue* would flow through my mind again and again. Little did I know how desperately I would need the Lord's rescue in the days ahead.

Another song often sung by a young woman in our church is, *Lay it Down*. It speaks of the importance of just laying out our cares before the Lord and giving them to him. It stresses how we become exhausted with the things in life and all we can do is give those things to the Lord. How could I know that this was exactly what I would need to do in the days ahead, do like I had never done before?

And then there were the southern gospel songs that anchored the "Singing Robbins" repertoire, "Farther along, we'll know all about it. Farther along, we'll understand why. Cheer up my

23

brother. Live in the sunshine. We'll understand it all by and by."
Or, "Precious Lord, take my hand. Lead me on. Let me stand."
How badly I would need the Lord to take my hand during the
situation I would be facing. I am so grateful for the reality of
Jehovah Jireh!

Tuesday evening, November 15, I left the Cancer Center
room of Helen Garber and went home to rest. Wednesday I felt
horrible. I stayed in bed most of the next two days. It was on
Thursday that I determined to see a doctor. The experience of the
collapse I had experienced after shooting the deer continued to
haunt me. I kept wondering if I had experienced a stroke or mild
heart attack. I became convinced something serious was going
on.

I set an appointment to see a doctor on November 18. That
appointment became my "ultimate stretch." I'll explain.

Chapter 3
The Ultimate Stretch

For me, November 18, 2005 was D-day for the most difficult time I've ever experienced. It was the beginning of what I call The Ultimate Stretch. I'm referring primarily to being stretched spiritually, those difficult times when God allows the unthinkable to occur in order to increase our spiritual capacity. Sometimes it seems like God just takes us and pulls in every direction, the same way we would pull on a rubber band. He pulls this way, and then that way, until we feel like we're being pulled in two and our band is going to break. Then he releases us, and in our relief, we find the process of stretching has increased our spiritual and moral capacity.

Through many sermons, I've talked to my congregation about God's stretching process. I've found he often uses prolonged circumstances— trials, heartaches, and painful problems—to stretch and enlarge our capacity, the capacity to be patient, merciful, compassionate, and long-suffering. He uses these experiences as a means to fully germinate the "fruit of the Spirit" within our lives. Looking back on the early years of my ministry, I can see that my capacity was increased many times through this stretching process. The book of James puts a capstone to this process by saying:

> *Consider it pure joy when you go through trials of various kinds.*

Wow! Joy from trials. Stretching that strengthens us. Difficulties designed for our good. It's true; some of the hardest experiences I've lived through—nervous breakdowns, tragedies involving our sons, confronting a life threatening illness—have become some of the best experiences of my life. I'm not saying they were easy or enjoyable. But I am saying they were transformational. They helped me grow significantly and mature exponentially. I find myself grateful to a God who cares enough to mold and shape us into the persons he wants us to be.

The Bible says that the teaching of the cross is foolishness to the world around us. Confronting a life threatening illness and calling it a good experience will also sound like foolishness. However, I can honestly say, from the bottom of my heart, that **if I could roll back time, I would not change one single part of my experience.** It was incredibly valuable in developing me and enlarging my spiritual capacity.

There is a lot of distorted teaching within religious circles regarding trials, suffering, and difficulties as related to Christian living. Some only emphasize the blessings, the wonderful things that God is going to do. They claim health and wealth for all, painting a rosy picture of heaven-on-earth for following the Lord. Such teaching is not Scriptural. In the Gospel of John, Jesus said:

> *"In this world you will have tribulation, but be of good cheer. I have overcome the world."*

The English word tribulation comes from the Greek word *thlipsis*; it means pressures, trials, difficulties, and hardships. Jesus affirmed that, in the fallen world in which we live, tribulation—pressures, trials, difficulties, hardships—abounds. This is not what God originally intended. God made a beautiful world. The creation account in Genesis, the first book of the Bible, concludes each act of divine creation by quoting God as saying, *"It is good!"*

All creation, including mankind, was made perfect and flawless. In addition, God blessed mankind above all other creatures by giving it the power of choice. God wanted and

26

intended for man to live forever in a loving relationship with himself. But we know from Genesis, chapter 3, that mankind made a conscious choice to go another direction. Through the temptation of the serpent (Satan), and man's decision to disobey God's command, sin entered the world. God's perfect creation was marred and became marked by decay and death. Thus, we live in a fallen world, a world that is plagued by the curse of sin. To make matters worse, generation after generation has followed lockstep down the pathway of wrong choices.

The Bible says Satan is the god of this age, meaning he is the one mankind has chosen to follow. The Bible also says that in the age to come, there will be a new heaven and a new earth. The book of Revelation describes a place where the curse has been lifted, where tears, pain, and suffering no longer exist. But a 21st-century fallen world lives in a time of *thlipsis*—tribulation, pressure, trial, difficulty, and hardship. The good news is, we have someone to turn to. We have someone to lean upon. Psalm 23 says:

Even though I walk through the valley of the shadow of death I will fear no evil, for Thou art with me.

How wonderful it was for me to enter into what became the biggest stretch of my life, knowing God would be with me. For years, I had stood at bedsides and gravesides sharing scriptures and other encouraging words, assuring people that God would be with them in their difficulties. How reassuring to see God do the same for me in my hour of *thlipsis*. All that He says about the "peace that passes all understanding" is true. I can honestly say that the calmness the Lord promises was there in my hour of need.

For a couple of years prior to November 18, I had been challenging my congregation to go to the next level of spiritual maturity. I tried to help them fully understand what it means to be the mature people of God. I explained that I would have failed as their pastor if our church were just a social club or community gathering. My goal, in being their pastor, was to see them develop spiritually and produce the fruits of the spirit in abundance.

Three or four years before, I had read a book titled, *Hind's Feet in High Places* (a hind is a young deer that existed in Israel in Old Testament times). This book tells the story of a girl named Little Crippled Much Afraid, a precious little girl who would often look up into the mountains and see young deer leaping from rock to rock. Being crippled, she wished with all of her heart to be able to run and jump like the deer. Her dream was to have feet like a hind, and masterfully conquer the mountainous terrain, no matter how high or difficult it might be.

The book tells how, in her own special way, she "climbed the mountain," and how God developed her through the climbing process. Through that book and various Scriptures, God challenged me to go to the next spiritual level in my own life, to move forward and set a pace for the church he had given me to shepherd. Since I believe followers can be limited by the capacity of their leaders, I knew that if I kept stretching and enlarging my capacity, my congregation would follow suit. They would grow as I prayed for them and lead by example.

While in the midst of reading this book, Jerry Hinds, the younger sibling of Dave Hinds, my brother-in-law, came to our church. Facing cancer and all the difficulties that accompany that dreaded disease, he challenged us with his tremendous faith. I often heard him refer to the doctor he had in Indianapolis, a physician I'll be referring to later, as very special man. Jerry went to be with the Lord about six months after he spoke at our church. I helped officiate at his funeral in Marion, Indiana, and sang one of his favorite songs, *Give Me Jesus.* He loved the final verse:

28

When I come to die . . .
        When I come to die, give me Jesus.
        You can have all this world, but give me Jesus.

No matter what we own and no matter what our position in life may be, when it comes to facing death, all that matters is our relationship with Jesus. It's not religious affiliation or church membership; it is about our relationship with Jesus Christ.

A number of years ago I visited an older woman who was close to death. As I leaned close to her ear I softly asked, "Do you know the Lord?"

She quickly responded, "I've been a Methodist for 30 years."

I softly replied, "Ma'am, that's not what I asked you."

With all the respect she was due, I had to say and emphasize that knowing the Lord was the important thing.

For a couple of years, I had been challenging the congregation to pursue the next spiritual level. How humbling it was to see people step forward and seek deeper spiritual commitment. Three years earlier, I had preached a sermon on the martyrs described in the book of Revelation. The main point of my message was that the highest commitment we can make to God is the martyr's commitment, that we may never be asked to die for our faith, but God wants us to make that level of commitment.

At the end of the sermon, and with head bowed, I asked if anyone would want to come forward, kneel at the altar, and acknowledge their desire to make a martyr's commitment. I thought five or ten people out of the 300 present might come forward. Hearing the rustle of feet, I opened my eyes and looked up to see three fourths of the congregation moving to the front, kneeling at the altar, and filling the surrounding aisles on their knees. I cried with joy! I realized we were people who wanted to go to the next spiritual level.

However, the next level comes as a process and with a price. That is what stretching is all about. And my ultimate stretch began November 18, 2005. As I said in the previous chapter, I'd been feeling sick, with severe bouts of weakness and dizziness. Thinking I had the flu, I expected my illness to run its course and leave me stronger than ever. By Thursday, November 17, no relief was in sight, my symptoms were worse, and I strongly suspected there was more wrong with me than a severe case of the flu. Haunted by the experience of collapsing while hunting, I sought medical help. My wife went with me to Dr. Savage's office, a local physician in Peru, Indiana, seven or eight miles from our home. Since the doctor wasn't there that morning, I saw the nurse practitioner, Josephine Estes, a lady I knew from the hospital where she worked and where I often made ministerial visits. I recited all of my symptoms for her and said I wanted to get to the bottom of this problem, and asked her for a comprehensive examination. Jo and her medical colleagues drew some blood, took some x-rays, and ran a number of tests. Though I still felt dizzy, we headed for home. All I wanted to do was rest. While my wife went back to work at the church, I stretched out on the couch, and laid the phone near my head in case I received any calls.

Sure enough, the phone rang. I looked at the ID and it said Dr. Savage's office. I answered the phone, and an emphatic voice at the other end said, "This is Dr. Savage's office. We need you to come back to our office immediately!" I replied that I would come as soon as possible, realizing that something must be seriously wrong. Still feeling dizzy and figuring I probably shouldn't drive by myself, I paged my accountability partner, Mark Hartinger, hoping he would call back immediately and then take me to Dr. Savage's office. (Mark is an anesthetist at the local hospital, so I didn't know if he would be available.) I called my wife at the church and told her I was going back to the doctor's office and that Mark would probably be going with me. I waited several minutes for Mark to call. When no call came, I walked out to my truck deciding to drive myself to the doctor's office.

I'll never forget getting into my truck with an acute awareness that something pretty serious was probably wrong with me. I remember sitting there with bowed head praying, "Lord, we've preached together; we've sung together; we've rode horses together. Heaven knows we've hunted together. Thank you for being my friend. Now I need you to go with me to the doctor's office. Amen."

I started down the driveway with no idea how Jehovah Jireh (the God who sees ahead and provides) would answer my prayer. But I had asked Him to go with me and I knew he was right alongside. As I drove out of the driveway, I saw Mark coming down the road. He pulled up beside me, rolled down his window and asked,

"Where are you going?"

I said, "I'm going to the doctor's office. Why are you here?"

He answered, "When you paged me, rather than call back, something told me to come—to come here to your home."

I've often been struck with awe at how God cares for every detail of our life. And, I need to pause for a moment, and comment on those details. The first sermon I ever preached as a young man (I'm sure it wasn't a very good sermon) was from the book of Proverbs where it says:

> *"Acknowledge the Lord in all of your ways, and He will direct your paths."*

That verse gripped me. I read it to mean that if I only acknowledged the Lord in a few areas of my life, and only talked to Him occasionally, those were the only areas where I would sense His direction. But if I cultivated a close friendship with him as Moses, the "friend of God" did, acknowledged him in all of the areas of my life, and talked to Him constantly about all of the details of my life, I would see his hand at work, right down to the smallest detail. He would go hunting with me; he would ride horses with me; and his presence would be with me while driving down the highway to a doctor's office. As the Scripture says,

"He is a friend who sticks closer than a brother."

I took my vehicle back to the house, got into Mark's truck, and headed for the doctor's office. As I entered the office, I could tell that Dr. Savage, who had returned for afternoon hours, was very nervous about talking to me. Even though he was a well-trained, professional man who deals with illness constantly, he seemed very ill at ease. He began asking general questions like, "How long have you felt bad?" I wondered if he was just making conversation because he didn't seem to want to say what apparently needed to be said.

Finally, he sat down, looked me straight in the eye, and said, "Tom, I have some bad news for you. You have leukemia. These test results can be nothing but leukemia. Your blood test shows your white cell count at 137,000." (White cell count in a normal, healthy male ranges from 5,000 to 11,000.) He went on to say, "An accelerated white cell count can be caused by a blood infection, but if you had an infection this severe, you would be dead. This can be nothing other than leukemia. We need to get you to a specialist as soon as possible since we do not have the capacity here at the local hospital to deal with numbers this high." Then he said, "In all my years of medical practice, I have never seen a white cell count this high." (Since then, I have learned that other leukemia patients can have similar high counts. However, his obvious point was to emphasize that my white cell count was extremely and dangerously high.) As we sat there for several minutes, I became aware that, though the test results were startling, there was a serene calmness both within me, and surrounding me. I suspect my serenity shocked him. I would like to ask Dr. Savage about it sometime in the future.

Finally, I looked back at him and said, "Well, what do we need to do?"

He said, "You need to pick a specialist. I'll give you a couple of choices." He began naming various specialists, and when he came to the name Dr. Becker, something inside said, "Becker. Becker." I cannot explain my inner resonance with that name other than I believe it was the prompting of the Holy Spirit. So I told him I preferred Dr. Becker. Since it was a Friday, Dr. Savage made an appointment with Dr. Becker for Monday morning and sent me home.

Since that time, numerous medical experts have told me they could not believe the doctor sent me home. They feel I should have been placed in an ambulance and taken to a large, high-tech facility for immediate treatment. I'll always believe that what Dr. Savage did, though unusual, was God ordered, because it was exactly what I needed. As I mentioned earlier, I had tried to develop a strong prayer life. Every problem, regardless of its size, I had taken to the Lord. As a result, I had developed a strong discomfort for quick decisions and hasty actions. I needed to think through things. I needed to pray about them.

It was very important to me to handle such a critical matter with my family and my church in an appropriate way. Because God knows us better than common sense may always dictate, I believe he led the doctor to send me home, even though it may have been a questionable thing to do. I'll always be grateful for Dr. Savage's course of action.

Mark took me home to an empty house. I sensed that Mark felt he needed to stay with me. I remember standing in the driveway asking him to please feel free to leave, for I needed to be alone. I needed time to pray. I needed time to adjust to this new reality. I needed a couple hours alone with God before my wife came home. I asked Mark to please trust me, and he responded positively with tears in his eyes. I will always appreciate the way this dear friend honored my request, putting aside his own informed medical opinion, and acquiescing to the deepest desires of my heart. He reluctantly but graciously drove away.

I entered the house and began to walk from room to room, for I walk when I pray. As I began pacing back and forth, I remember praying a very simple, child-like, straight-to-the-point prayer, "Lord, I've got leukemia and I need your help." Almost immediately I sensed his presence. Our God, a help in time of trouble, was very present.

Years ago, hymn writer Thomas Chisholm penned these comforting words:

> Great is thy faithfulness, O God, my Father.
> There is no shadow of turning with thee.
> Thou changest not. Thy compassions, they fail not.
> As thou hast been, thou forever wilt be.
> Great is thy faithfulness.
> Great is thy faithfulness.
> Morning by morning, new mercies I see.
> All I have needed, thy hand hath provided.
> Great is thy faithfulness, Lord unto me.

I found, in that beginning moment of the ultimate stretch, the generous grace and comfort God gives when we face a difficult future. As I prayed for the next hour or so, a divine calmness enveloped me to such a degree that fear didn't have a chance. And I began to prepare myself for my wife's return.

I heard her pull into the driveway; words fail me to describe my feelings as I saw her little blue car coming up the lane. When she came in the house, her very first question was, "What did you find out at the doctor's office?" I remember putting both of my arms around her, looking her in the eye, and saying, "Pam, I've got leukemia." We stood at the kitchen counter for the longest time, with our arms around each other, saying nothing. We had been married 30 years, and at that point, we had already gone through a number of deep valleys together. So, we just stood there and cried, grateful that God was nearby and we were still together.

That evening I called three of our sons, Scott, Allen, and Kevin, students at the Christ for the Nations school in Dallas, Texas, to personally tell them the news. Our oldest son, Tom, a high school varsity girls' basketball coach, had a game that evening, and I didn't want him to know about my leukemia until the game was over. After the game, Pam and I drove to his home and told him the news. While Scott, Allen, and Kevin had seemed to accept the news fairly well, I could see that Tom was strongly disturbed. He was hard to read. I'll explain more about this in the next chapter.

We left and headed home. My symptoms intensified. I had begun bleeding between my teeth—blood spots in my mouth; blood slowly oozing from my nose; red spots all over my legs (petechiae, caused by the bursting of small capillaries). I remember going to bed wondering if I would wake up. While Dr. Savage wasn't a leukemia specialist, he did warn me that my elevated white cell count could produce severe hemorrhaging, and I was hemorrhaging. Here I was, stretched out on the bed, knowing my body was in the process of destroying itself, oozing blood, while enveloped by peace, an inner, incredible contentment. Though I was fully aware I could die in my sleep, I wasn't afraid. In fact, I had a twinge of excitement, as strange as it may seem, that I might see the Lord before the night was over. And, I knew in my heart that I was ready to meet him.

There's something else I need to say. It's so much easier to face death knowing, without a shadow of a doubt, that there's nothing you need to straighten out with another person. I've often heard of individuals, who's first thought when facing death was,

"I have to straighten out a situation with my brother."

"I must talk to someone with whom I've been malicious."

"I need to work out some ill feelings with my father."

"I must go to my employer and confess some sin."

What a wonderful feeling to go to bed that night with the assurance my slate was clear and there was nothing to straighten out. That's not a statement about perfection for I've made many mistakes as a husband, father, and pastor. I'm thankful God doesn't call us to be perfect. But he does call us to be faithful.

In the King James translation of the Bible, there is a verse in the Sermon on the Mount that says, *"Be ye therefore perfect as your Father in heaven is perfect."* The word *perfect* can be translated as *complete.* Because the Christian life is a process, God wants to move us toward completion, toward full spiritual maturity. This takes time, often many years, and a lot of stretching. Thus, while we're not perfect, we can be faithful to the process. How grateful I was, at that late Friday night hour, to relax in the spiritual discipline of faithfulness. I seemed to have only one concern, and before I went to sleep, I asked God to shield my wife from anything that would be painful for her. I was not afraid of leaving this world, but I was concerned that, if serious hemorrhaging occurred during the night, my wife would be left with a very bad memory.

I awoke the next morning happy to be alive. A near-death encounter is a very valuable experience. As someone once said, "You've never really lived until you've nearly died." Saturday morning, in new and fresh ways, I sat, coffee cup in hand, savoring the simpler things of life: the view of our distant woods; a second cup of hot coffee; the closeness of someone you dearly love. I was blest, indeed! Throughout the night, I had given some thought to what I needed to do on this second day of the ultimate stretch, for I wanted to handle my new reality in a manner consistent with my call to faithful ministry. I wanted to honor the Lord in all things, and be a leader who, regardless of whether things went well or not, made good decisions and set a good example. I remember praying, "Lord, give me skill in handling this situation. Help me to fulfill my responsibility with excellence."

I began making phone calls, inviting our church leaders to come to our home so I could tell them my news. I called our assistant pastor, Chris Edgington, and asked him to handle the Sunday services. Because we have so many new believers in our congregation, I felt it would be premature to share my condition with everyone until a leukemia specialist could confirm my diagnosis. So I asked Chris to tell the congregation that I was ill and requested their prayers. It encouraged me to realize, that through the fever, dizziness, and weakness of the weekend, God had given me the wisdom to fulfill my responsibility. He knew and fulfilled the desire of my heart. Matthew 6:33 says:

> *Seek ye first the kingdom of God and His righteousness and he'll add everything to you.*

I've found that if you put God's will and work ahead of other matters, he will take care of everything else. Since then, many have asked, "By not going to a hospital immediately, couldn't you have died over the weekend?" Medically speaking, the answer is yes. But I believe my steps were "ordered of the Lord," and he wanted me to spend the weekend at home so I could properly care for my flock. He, who laid down his life for the sheep, sets a high bar for shepherds. I wanted to be counted among those called good shepherds. To allow others to call you a pastor and not be a good shepherd is totally incongruous. I've not always been the best shepherd, but my heart's desire was to be stretched to a greater capacity for effective shepherding.

I spent the balance of Saturday meeting with church leaders and sharing my condition with them. I'll never forget how Bryan Jaberg, my faithful prayer partner, bent down over me as I was lying on the floor, and petitioned the throne of grace for my healing. It was one of those very special prayer moments, a moment that helped me make it through an exhausting day with a feeling I had accomplished everything that needed to be done.

I knew that Jehovah Jireh, the God who sees ahead, was at work, but I couldn't see much beyond Saturday. This surprised me for I almost always have a sense of how things will go. I'm not sure how or why this happens; I've always felt it came from the Holy Spirit as part of the gift of shepherding. I was mystified, as I candidly shared with my church leaders, that I didn't know where this new reality was going to take us.

Various leaders very carefully asked,

"Tom, how do you think this will turn out?"

I said all I knew to say, "I don't know. It may be my time to die."

I wasn't disturbed by their question, but I was distressed that the immediate future of the church's ministry might be affected by my medical condition, and, contrary to other times, I didn't have the faintest idea of what the next step ought to be. I wasn't feeling totally competent as a shepherd.

Still disturbed, I determined to take a prayer walk Sunday morning. Given my medical condition, some may have thought it foolish to do so, but I felt impressed to do what I had always done. I thought of Daniel, who threw open his window and prayed towards Jerusalem, as he had always done, even though his prayers resulted in his being thrown into a den of lions. Because I believed and taught that faithfulness to God must not be affected by circumstances or disturbances of any kind, I needed to practice what I preached.

I also called my brother Jim, a pastor in Van Wert, Ohio, and asked if he and his wife Helen would join me at the church, around 3:00 p.m., for a special time of prayer. In keeping with scripture, I wanted to be anointed and prayed for by Jim and some of our church leaders before I met with the leukemia specialist Monday morning. After prayer and much thought, I asked a handful of relatives and very close, long-time friends to gather for this special service. The group included my other prayer partner, Dave Hinds and his wife, Kathy. Dave, Kathy, along with Pam's parents, Max and Luella came to our home about 2:00 p.m. so we could ride together to the church for the prayer service.

While the whole day was ordered of the Lord, I had no idea of how significant that hour between 2:00 p.m. and 3:00 p.m. with Kathy and Dave would become.

Chapter 4

A Word from the Lord ... My Three Requests

How sweet it is to receive a definite word from the Lord! His word came Sunday, November 20, through a very faithful servant, my sister-in-law, Kathy Hinds.

This Biblical phrase, "a word from the Lord," is often misused in today's religious culture. Improperly used, it can mean anything from a certain impulsive feeling to a distorted, misleading fact. Properly used, it can mean the application of Holy Scripture to a particular situation. We believe that the Bible is God's inspired Word - "All Scripture is given by inspiration of God," the Bible says. I have found, as have so many others, God will speak to you very specifically from His Word when you need His guidance. You'll know in your heart of hearts, without any question, that a specific passage of Scripture is speaking to you. This can happen while reading His Word or can come through another person who knows His Word. I've had times in my life when someone would come to me and say something, totally unaware that they were being used by God to give me something from Him.

One may ask, "How do you know it's a word from the Lord?"

While preaching, I've asked my congregation, "How do you know your mother is your mother? Certainly you have a birth certificate. Certainly you carry her identity. But, that's not how you know. Proof comes from your heart of hearts. You know your mother is your mother because of how she has related to you, how she has communicated with you while raising you; those times of sickness when you were burning up with fever and she held you close; those times when she protected you and looked after you. Through that love, compassion, and tenderness, in a variety of circumstances, she somehow communicated to your heart. You knew she was your mother."

This is an excellent example of how we know God, how we know His voice. As we walk life's pathway with the Lord, through the valleys of affliction and difficulty, God tenderly helps us, leads us, and comforts us. We develop a growing awareness deep within us that He is God; that we are His. We begin to recognize and understand His voice. As Jesus said, "My sheep know my voice."

After my four sons were born, I saw them begin to develop one by one. Even as babies, they could recognize my voice in a room. While they didn't always understand what I was saying, as they grew and we spent time together, they not only recognized my voice, they began to understand my voice and know me. And so it is with the Lord.

Kathy and her husband Dave came over to our house on that particular Sunday, and before we left for church she said she wanted to share some Scripture that God had given her for me. This was somewhat out of character for Kathy, so it caught my attention. She proceeded to read from II Kings, chapter 20:

> *In those days Hezekiah became ill and was at the point of death. And the prophet Isaiah went unto him and said, "This is what the Lord says: 'Put your house in order because you are going to die. You will not recover.'"*
>
> *Hezekiah turned his face to the wall and prayed to the Lord, "Remember, O Lord, how I have walked before you faithfully, and with whole-hearted devotion have done what is good in your sight." And Hezekiah wept bitterly.*

41

At this point in her reading, Kathy began to sob and cry. Those of us in the room with her were deeply moved and began to cry with her. After collecting herself, she continued to read:

> *Before Isaiah had left the middle court, the word of the Lord came to him, "Go back and tell Hezekiah, the leader of my people, this is what the Lord, the God of your father, David, says, 'I have heard your prayer and seen your tears, and I will heal you. And on the third day from now you will go up to the temple, and I will add 15 years to your life.'"*

I was stunned by these verses. I can't express how much I wanted to believe that what she read applied to me. But I knew, in a life and death situation, it would only be normal for me to reach out and grasp some Biblical passage for hope and assurance. Since it was nearing 3:00 p.m., and feeling the time pressure to leave for the church, we spent a few moments in prayer in our living room, got in our vehicles and proceeded to the church where I was to be anointed.

It's interesting to note that in the II Kings 20:1-6 passage it says, "You will go up to the temple on the third day." I didn't realize until later that I was going up to the church to be anointed on the third day. On Friday the 18th, the first day, I had found out about my leukemia; on Saturday the 19th, the second day, I met with our church leaders; and on Sunday the 20th, the third day, I was "going up" to the church to be anointed! It's interesting that God, when He gives you "a word from the Lord," attends to the smallest of details.

It's also interesting to note that before Kathy read this passage for me, I had felt compelled to go to the church to be anointed. Given how exhausted I was feeling, my wife had strongly suggested I might invite everyone to come to our house for prayer and the anointing. While her suggestion made perfect sense, I was insistent about going to the church. At the time, I thought it was because the church meant so much to me and was the place where I ministered. Looking back, I believe God was showing me how perfectly He would give His word to me through Scripture.

I never will forget walking into the church that day. As I approached the walkway and opened the door, my most trusted friends, including my sister Miriam, her husband Jesse, and my brother Jim and his wife, Helen, greeted me. I asked the group to gather around the altar, saying I would join them after a quick restroom stop. I wanted to look in a mirror to check my teeth before going up front and praying with them. On and off, throughout the weekend, I had begun to bleed between my teeth, as well as from my nose. Bleeding had started again that Sunday, and I felt seeing it might be difficult for some of them. As I went to the front, I found a place to sit right in the middle of my group of friends, planning to ask my older brother, Jim, to anoint and pray for me.

I'd like to pause for a moment and talk about my brother. I have two excellent brothers. My oldest brother, Paul, lives in the Chicago area. He was 19 years old and had left home for college before I was born, so we didn't spend much time together. I value him very much and have appreciated his input into my life through the years.

Jim, on the other hand, was 16 and living at home. Due to the absence caused by my father's itinerant ministry, Jim became a father figure for me. I've been teased many times by him about how he cared for me, changed my diapers, and gave me my baths. Now, years later, we're both pastors. It doesn't seem to me we're 16 years apart in age. I still feel very close to him. Jim probably exemplifies a servant's heart more than anyone I know.

Some years ago, he helped me put a roof on my father's mobile home. Jim, who knows very little about construction, roofing, or building of any kind, came to me in a most humble way, and said, "Tom, you are so much better at this than me. Rather than you trying to show me how to roof, why don't I be the one who carries the shingles, hands you the tools, and helps you with whatever needs to be done?" This attitude is a window into Jim's heart. Here I was, his kid brother, being asked to let him serve me! Seeing this spirit of Christ in Jim drew me toward wanting him to be the one to anoint and pray for me. The scripture says:

Let the greatest among you be the servant.

Prior to the prayer, I asked if I could open my heart to them for a few minutes and share three requests. At that time, I didn't realize how important these requests were, including the order in which I gave them. I was only following the deepest thoughts of my heart. I recall saying somewhat vividly, "I have three requests. I'm going to give them to you in order of importance, beginning with the least important. The third and least important request is, please pray that, *if God so wills, he would touch my body.* The second request, somewhat more important, is that *He would dissolve my fears.* The reason I request prayer about fear is because I have visited cancer patients for years, and I am very aware of the kind of suffering cancer can bring and what that suffering can do to a person. The devil is harassing me with fearful thoughts. Pray that my fears will be dissolved."

And then I said, "My main request, which is most important to me, is to ask you to pray that, no matter what happens, *I will suffer honorably.*" I went on to explain: "Nothing is more disheartening to a congregation than holding someone in high esteem spiritually, respecting them for their spiritual leadership, and then, when the pressure is on, seeing them buckle. We have all seen this happen at times and have been inwardly

44

disappointed. I'm aware that many people may look up to me as an example, especially young people and new believers. And I don't know what I may be called to suffer. But through that suffering, my desire is to be Christ-like in my attitudes, be grateful to the doctors and nurses, people ministering to me, and demonstrate the spirit of Christ-to suffer honorably. That is my most important request." I can truly say if there ever was a statement from my heart, that request was from my heart. With the sharing of my requests, my friends and family knelt around me, and I handed my brother a bottle of anointing oil.

I need to take a moment to talk about anointing oil. I have two bottles of anointing oil (olive oil). One I keep on a shelf in my bedroom at home and the other one I keep in my briefcase. The one on the shelf, I used to anoint my mother for healing. But she passed away. I have accepted God's decision. I believe it was God's time for her to go. I also used that same oil to anoint Barbara Troyer and Linda Swetnam. God called both Barbara and Linda home. Like my mother, their healing came through gloriously new bodies, beautifully restored in heaven. While I believe physical healing is provided in Christ's atonement, healing can be a matter of timing. The scriptures say, "Through His stripes we are healed" (Isaiah 53). We pray. We anoint. We trust. Timing is up to the Lord.

As I passed the bottle to Jim, I was aware that before we came to the church, I had gone into the bedroom to retrieve the oil that had anointed Mom, Barbara and Linda. As I took it from a shelf something said to me as clear as can be, "Don't take that oil. You're not going to die." As a result of that voice, I took the small bottle from my briefcase. So at the church, when it was time for Jim to pray, I handed him the small bottle from my briefcase. The group was unaware of my experience.

I don't remember all of the words of Jim's prayer, but I'll never forget the spirit of his prayer, as he cried and prayed with the

45

earnestness of a child talking to his father. He asked God to touch me, His servant, and anointed me with oil. We completed our prayer time and I hugged everyone in the group. Pam and I went to our vehicle and drove home. I found myself very much at peace. A God-like calmness was with me though I was conscious of entering into a time of great travail. As I went to bed that evening, I had a keen awareness that this could be my last night on earth. But, again, I felt the comfort of the Holy Spirit.

I'd like to share my thoughts about the Holy Spirit. We live in an era when there is a lot of talk about the Holy Spirit-lots of viewpoints about who He is, what He does, and how He manifests Himself. It's always been interesting to me that when Jesus introduced the Holy Spirit to His disciples, and explained that the Holy Spirit was coming into the world, Jesus called Him the Comforter (John 14).

I believe the primary ministry of the Holy Spirit is to comfort us. One of the deepest needs of the human heart is the need for comfort. Often when people seek pleasure, success, or intimate relationships, what they're really looking for is comfort and assurance. This is why God is so patient, kind, and forgiving when we've become sinful and err in our pursuits. The Holy Spirit is the Comforter, the one who encourages and strengthens. I also believe that a true sign of whether we're filled with the Holy Spirit is our desire and ability to comfort and encourage others, since that's His primary ministry.

Pam and I went to sleep that night, and my mind drifted to the verses in II Kings 20 that Kathy had given me. Around 4:00 a.m., God began drawing me toward reading those verses for myself. I needed to know in my heart of hearts if those verses were for me.

Through the years, I've seen many people grab onto a verse (usually out of context) and claim it as God's promise for them. I often wondered if that verse really was for them or if they were grasping for straws of hope, something to hang onto. At the same time, I've always believed God will confirm His promises again and again when those promises are unquestionably for you.

With that belief in mind, I sat in the corner recliner, and opened my Bible to II Kings. In the darkness and stillness of that early morning hour, with a small light shining over my Bible, I said, "Lord, I'm preparing to go to an oncology specialist today. I'm sure I'll be hospitalized. I don't know what the future holds. I need to know. Are those verses Kathy read verses that apply to me?"

I began reading through the verses. When I came to the one that read, "I will heal you," I began sobbing. It is not uncommon for me to cry during my time with the Lord, but this was unusual. I felt in my heart of hearts an incredible sense of God's presence in that dark and quiet room. I was reminded of the question I had often asked my congregation, "How do you know your mother is your mother?" and the answer I often gave, "It's how she communicated to your heart that made you positive, with no shadow of doubt."

I knew, then and there, in my heart of hearts, those verses were for me. They were a "word from the Lord," I could claim for my future!

My wife got up a little bit later, and I shared with her how God had assured me through his Word and His presence. She, in turn, shared with me a Scripture that God had brought to her attention:

> *"I'll be with him in trouble. He will call me and I will answer him. I will deliver him. With long life I will satisfy him and show him my salvation"* Psalm 91.

47

Before we left for the oncologist's office, I felt I should call my son, Tom. As I said previously, Tom had struggled tremendously with the news of my leukemia the past Friday evening. And I wasn't totally sure what his unusual quietness indicated. I called him by phone and told him that God had prompted me to call him though I didn't know why. I read to him the passage from II Kings and told him that God had clearly confirmed to me that he was going to heal me and add 15 years to my life.

I could sense an immediate change in his spirit. Later I found out Tom had experienced very alarming feelings about my leukemia through the weekend. He had even made the statement, "I don't feel good about this. I think we're going to lose my Dad."

Here again, we see God's faithfulness to every member of the family. And these words I'm writing can never express how undeserving I am of all this faithfulness. It is important to say that God's faithfulness has nothing to do with me being a minister. It has nothing to do with any goodness of my own. I have found God to be equally faithful to every believer who truly decides to follow him. He is no respecter of persons. He doesn't favor pastors over lay people. He doesn't favor the famous or "important" people over the unknown or everyday people. I only wish everyone would choose to follow Him so they could experience His faithfulness.

It was Monday, the 21st, time to consult with the oncologist. We got in our vehicle and drove to Dr. Becker's office in Kokomo. While I had been given directions, I didn't recall ever being there before. But, as we approached the building and pulled into the parking lot, I realized that it was the same building where I had visited with the Garbers the Tuesday before. Here again, I saw God preparing me for what was to come.

As we entered the lobby, I showed my wife the place where I had sat and visited with the Garbers. Only then did I realize that Dr. Becker was her doctor. I was intrigued that I had been impressed to choose Dr. Becker, unaware that she was so fond of him.

After some additional blood tests, Dr. Becker and an intern from the Indiana University Medical Center in Indianapolis took me into a small conference room for a conversation I'll never forget as long as I live. He began by giving me a tape recorder and setting it to record. He said it was customary to tape these conversations because they tended to be very intense and emotional. Sometimes the emotion of the moment blocked the patient's ability to hear what was being said. By taping the conversation, the patient could listen to the tape again at a later time. The recorder only confirmed in my mind that I was about to engage in one of the most critical conversations I'd ever been in.

Dr. Becker got to the point quickly. He began by saying that I was a medical emergency. I was much worse shape than the doctor in my hometown of Peru had believed and I had two hours to make a decision about ongoing treatment. He said he couldn't believe I hadn't brain-hemorrhaged by now for my blood test of a few minutes before registered a dangerously high white count of 137,000, as compared to a normal, healthy white count of between 5,000 and 11,000.

He paused and gave me just a little time to adjust to what he said. Feeling confused and unsure of myself I responded, "So, what do I do?" In my mind I was thinking, I'll go home, get some clothes together, and we will drive to whatever hospital he suggests for treatment. With some urgency he said, "You need to be immediately transported to Indiana University Medical Center in Indianapolis. They have teams of leukemia specialists, including bone marrow transplant specialists."

49

I was taken aback by the thought of going to the IU Med Center. I knew hundreds of people had received tremendous help there, but I didn't want to go there. I had visited patients there in their glass cubicles, surrounded by all kinds of imposing machines. Though it is a fine hospital, it is also a training facility. I knew I would be seen by a variety of different doctors and interns. I had often said to my wife that I would prefer never to go there for treatment of any kind.

Again, I sensed God's faithfulness to me as a voice inside of me kept saying, "St. Vincent. St. Vincent. St. Vincent." I have always liked St. Vincent Hospital in Indianapolis, and I told my wife a number of years ago that if I was ever too sick to make my own decisions and had to be taken to a large hospital for specialized care, I would like to go to St. Vincent. So I asked Dr. Becker if I could say something. He said, "Sure."

I said, "Dr. Becker, I'm a simple man. I've been a pastor for 23 years. I've walked with the Lord for 31 years. I have always believed in an inner voice. I believe that your suggestion of IU Med Center, medically speaking, is a very good suggestion. I'm sure it's an excellent facility. But an inner voice keeps saying to me, "St. Vincent." As I began to cry, Dr. Becker came across the room, put his arms around me (which a doctor seldom does), and said, "If you hear an inner voice, you need to follow that voice. I've always believed in an inner voice." I sobbed pretty hard. I then told him I had a request. I said, "I know I need to go somewhere immediately. I accept your counsel. I understand I don't get to go home. I accept your directive. But, I am a man that needs time to adjust to things and to pray. May I go to the parking lot with my wife and walk and pray for half an hour before I leave?" In light of the urgency of his previous statements, I fully expected him to say no. However, his answer was, "Yes, you may, but don't leave the property." I'll always be appreciative to Dr. Becker for that kindness.

50

I also asked if I could call a physician friend, a prayer partner, to transport us to the hospital instead of going by ambulance. I knew that with the danger of eminent hemorrhaging, I did not want to be in a situation of just Pam and me in our own car. I also knew that if we went by ambulance, Pam might not be allowed to go with me. Again he made an exception and said that it would be okay. So I called my friend, Cathy Reese, and asked if she would come and take us to St Vincent hospital. She said she would be there very quickly. I found out later that she had turned her patients over to her partner and took the afternoon off in order to transport me to Indianapolis.

While we waited on Cathy, my wife and I walked around outside. We cried and hugged and prayed. What a precious time! What a special time to adjust to this new medical reality while sensing the presence of the Comforter. When Cathy arrived, we, along with our paperwork, got in her car, and headed for St. Vincent. I had made the trip to St. Vincent Hospital many times to visit patients. Now I was a patient.

Every pastor should be a patient. Though I had never been a patient in a hospital, I had visited hundreds of people in the hospital over the years. I had told them of God's goodness. I had read Scripture to encourage them at their bedside. But I never understood until that day what it really meant to be a patient. As a pastor, it can become routine to go to a hospital and visit with people who have just heard the most shocking news of their life and say, "God will be with you. You are safe in His hands." It's not routine when you are the person processing the shock. What a valuable experience! What a special privilege to discover that God was trusting me enough to allow me to suffer in order to identify with, and minister more effectively to His hurting flock. That is exactly how I view that day.

We arrived at the hospital and went to the admitting area. Again, how faithful God is - Jehovah Jireh, the one who provides and sees ahead. I sat down in the waiting room, and at eye level across from me on the wall was a portion of Psalm 23:

> *Yea, though I walk through the valley of the shadow of death, I will fear no evil, for Thou art with me.*

How faithful God is in every detail!

I was taken to my room on the "cancer floor," the sixth floor. Anyone who goes to St. Vincent dreads to be on the sixth floor. Little did I know I would be in a hospital room for 31 days without being able to leave its four walls. God gave me incredible grace during those days, which I'll share in the next few chapters.

I want to finish this chapter by saying my time in the hospital was a "day of visitation" in my life. What do I mean by that phrase? Let me put it this way. When you know Jesus Christ and walk with Him, you'll find that He is faithful to be with you, to watch over you, and to commune with you. But, there are special times, times I call a "day of visitation" when you experience something you recognize as highly unusual. In the next chapter I will elaborate on my "day of visitation." I preached a sermon in May of 2005 on this subject, five months before my leukemia was discovered. Isn't it incredible that I preached such a message, including references to cancer, five months before I knew I had it? Here again was God preparing the way.

Chapter 5
Day of Visitation

This chapter is somewhat of a parenthesis in my story. It paraphrases a sermon I preached on May 5, 2005, five months before discovering I had acute myeloid leukemia. I am placing the basic content of this sermon here because I want to explain the phrase "day of visitation," and why I believe my experience with leukemia was a day of visitation for me.

This morning I want to talk about what the Bible calls the "Day of Visitation." I would ask you to listen intently, with an open mind and heart.

What does the Bible mean by the "Day of Visitation?" It certainly must be an important occasion since it is specifically mentioned in Scripture some twelve to fourteen times. It's twin phrase, "Times of Visitation," appears numerous times in Scripture and is the same idea in a broader sense: God making Himself known to (visiting) us. But the "Day of Visitation" is much more specific and focused in nature. It is a specific, never to be forgotten, God-ordained experience which changes us, as well as how we live our lives. It is a "day" when God moves in very closely to us and tries to communicate with us about very specific matters.

Unfortunately, the day of visitation is not always recognized as such. In our preoccupation with a busy world, we, often and tragically, miss our day of visitation. We are cluttered with busy schedules and the accumulation of things that may not matter that much. We're overworked and tired. There's no time for reflection or meditation. No time to be quiet. No time to hear the "still small voice of God." And the clutter of life obscures and distorts any special visitation of God.

Are you listening? Are you guilty? We are talking about very serious, sobering matters—a personal visitation by God.

For those who are listening for God's voice, his day of visitation may begin with a trip to the funeral home. I do not know, nor do I profess to know or understand, all of the ways in which God works. His ways can be quite mysterious. I don't think you can chart them or graph them. I don't know why God moves so explicitly into my life at certain times and deals with me about personal matters in very specific ways and at very specific times. Why now? Why wasn't it a year ago? I don't know. What I do know is that, in my walk with the Lord, there have been numerous times when God has visited me in a very specific way through a variety of experiences and events.

I remember when I heard the news that my older sister, Carroll, had died. Though she was quite a bit older than me, we were very close. I often stayed with Carroll and her husband at their home in Marion, Indiana. Carroll had gone to the hospital for a simple D & C procedure. Not knowing she was allergic to the anesthetic, she suffered cardiac failure when it was given to her. At the time, I was a freshman in high school, involved in all kinds of things—on the debate team, making girlfriends, going a mile a minute.

But when I heard Carroll had died, it changed everything. I remember pacing back and forth in our family living room realizing nothing else really mattered at that moment. It didn't matter who became freshman class president. It didn't matter if this girl liked me or that girl liked me. Very suddenly, everything had changed.

It's easy to miss the day of visitation. It's easy to miss his voice as we traverse the mountaintops and valleys of life. As your pastor, may I open my heart to you? I have cried many,

54

many, times over people who I knew were missing their day of visitation. God was dealing very directly with them and they were oblivious to it. Thorns and weeds were choking the seed as Jesus said in the parable of the sower and the seed. God was trying to take the seed of His Word and prepare them for a wonderful and plenteous harvest, but the "cares of this life," the thorns, were choking the seed to extinction. They were spending their lives going in circles, accomplishing little, and reaping nothing. They were missing their day of visitation.

I'm not implying that as Christians we're hanging on to our salvation by the skin of our teeth. I'm not talking about heaven or hell. We are saved by grace through God's incredible mercy. Rather, I'm talking about spiritual growth. I'm talking about biblical discipleship. I'm talking about becoming everything God's wants us to be. I'm talking about the process of conforming to the image of God's Son, our Lord and Savior, Jesus Christ.

If you want to grow, you've got to be keen to those times when God visits you. And growth is often accompanied by pain, spiritual growing pains. Sometimes a visitation is announced by a crisis. Sometimes it's hearing the doctor in a soft, matter of fact way say, "You may have cancer." "What?" Cancer is one of the most terrifying words in the English language. But, if you are tuned to hear the voice of God, you may find cancer is a day of visitation.

Visitations can come in many different forms. I've seen times when family problems were a day of visitation, when God used a family crisis to help family members humble themselves before the Lord. Pam and I went through a family crisis with some of our children when I was pastoring at Chapel Hill. It was a time when God wanted to deal with me. He wanted to take me to another level. It was a crossroads time, for a day of visitation often begins at some kind of a crossroads. And, when visitations

55

occur, it's so easy to respond in angry, bitter ways. We can fume. We can fuss. We can say, "I'm not going to take it. I'm out of here." We can talk back to God: "What is this about? I never thought you would let this happen to me!"

Another form a day of visitation can take is chastisement—a day when God pulls you in and scolds you real well. I remember when a very godly man chastised me, and as I prayed about it, God spoke to me and said, "This is me, Tom! This is me!" Perhaps you are a person who is not setting the example that you should, and God pulls you in and chastises you. Remember, as the scripture says, "He chastises those he loves." It's because He cares about you the he visits you. Rather than rail angrily against him, we should be honored that the God of the universe would visit us so personally. Don't waste it. Don't take it lightly. Don't miss it.

While the Scriptures indicate that a day of visitation can be a time of chastisement or even judgment, I want to spend the rest of my time talking about how God uses a day of visitation as a golden opportunity to develop us, to take us to a higher level of relationship with Him. I had a day of visitation like this a few years ago. Maybe you can relate to my experience as I share it.

Seven and a half years ago Pam and I were in Chicago, where for the previous three years we had been involved in street ministry. During that time I had a nervous breakdown. I just fell apart. Looking back, there is no doubt in my mind that this nervous breakdown was a day of visitation for me, and it lasted for six long months.

How long is a time of visitation? It can be anything. The Scripture says a day with the Lord is like a thousand years and a thousand years is like one day. This is another way of saying, "Don't watch the clock." Rather, watch for the indicators that God is at work.

When ministers experience personal crisis, especially ones of long duration where the ministry itself comes to a screeching halt, it's so easy to say, "Lord, what's going on here? I'm your servant, working my heart out for you. Why are you letting this happen to me?" Even ministers can miss their day of visitation.

While in this time of nervous breakdown, I went to a Lake Michigan beach with my colleagues, Paul Moshesh and Jason Brannon, and through tears of confusion and discouragement I said, "I've just got to have some help with this street ministry. I'm falling apart and I don't know why. I don't understand this. I came to Chicago feeling I was led of the Lord to do street ministry. But it seems like I just can't do it. And to top it all off, the church I used to pastor seems to be struggling rather desperately ever since I left. I'm confused. I'm going through a time of deep despair and problems. I need help." And I cried and cried and cried.

As I struggled with the whole idea of a nervous breakdown, I remember thinking, "Mercy sakes, what should I do?" I talked to one of my overseers in the denomination where I was ordained, and he suggested that I might go back and get a job at the Kroger supermarket where I had been previously employed. It was like discussing my future with one of Job's friends. I went home and cried some more, praying, "Oh Lord, have I done so poorly that my former job is the only future option I have?"

But then, God began to deal with me. I stopped wondering if I was just helplessly caught in the vortex of one of life's many storms, and embraced my day of visitation. I started doubling my prayer time. Instead of walking and praying an hour a day, I started walking two or three hours a day, praying, "Lord, I'm listening to you. What do you want to say to me?" In those six months God spoke to me in ways I can't put into words. He changed me. He "grew" me. And that's why I was able to say to you when I came to this area to be your pastor, "I'm still fragile,

57

but if you will be patient with me, I think I can be a better pastor than I've ever been."

Chicago was my day of visitation—a time when God broke me down, helped me sort out my motives, refined my ministry commitment, and prepared me for a new level of effective ministry. In the meantime, I saw Paul Moshesh and Jason Brannon step up to the plate and help me expand our street ministry. And even in my time of deep brokenness, I was able to effectively mentor people in ministry.

So, what did I learn in Chicago? I learned to embrace the day of visitation, to let God work in my heart in a new way. I learned that failure and feelings of uselessness teach you lessons that can't be learned any other way. I learned to embrace the sorting of my motives, the refinement of my commitments, and I learned to swallow the divine medicine God provides for the toxic twins of envy and jealousy. I learned to trust Him to teach me what it means to have a broken heart and a tender spirit. I learned that He is faithful and desires the very best for me, even when everything around me says just the opposite.

I think some of you may be going through a time of visitation. If so, my prayer for you is, "Lord, don't let them miss what you are trying to say to them. They may feel like you are hurting them, or have abandoned them. They may be feeling pain they never have felt before, but it's their day of visitation. It's their time to step up to the plate and begin the journey to the new level you want for them."

My prayer partner, Bryan, stopped me before our worship service a few months ago for a quick hello. The moment I saw him, I knew something was seriously wrong. He gave me a hug and said he needed to talk to me. After the service he explained, "Tom, they told me I've got cancer." I don't know that this news was a day of visitation for my friend Bryan, but I suspect that it was. Only Bryan and God know for sure. What I do know is that his bout with cancer was life changing, the way a day of visitation can be life changing.

As I stand here in the pulpit this morning, I'm very conscious of a wonderful group of young people here on the first three rows. Would the rest of you mind if I speak directly to them for just a moment?

I believe that our recent Rally Team experiences were a day of visitation for some of you. Is it not true that we felt the hand of God upon us in an unusual way? I remember the pastor of Lakeview Wesleyan Church coming to me and saying, "Tom, I haven't felt God very many times like I felt Him this morning." Everywhere we went people said God touched them. Connie and Richard King are still talking about the day we came to their campground. They say they're still getting fruit from our ministry—people coming to them saying how our ministry touched their lives. I believe Rally Team was a day of visitation for many of you. Don't drift from it. Embrace what you learned. Make it part of your future.

May I share another personal story with all of you? It's about someone who may be passing up his day of visitation. I say this ever so cautiously; nevertheless, I believe it may be the case.

Pam and I were on our way back from Texas after visiting the college where our sons Scott, Allen, and Kevin were attending. We stopped at a motel for the night, and through a strange set of events, we become acquainted with the people who owned the place. It actually started when I sensed they were very wary of me. Apparently, we didn't match up to the usual customer profile. It's true; we were driving a borrowed truck, and asked to check out extra late (we were on vacation and wanted to relax for awhile). We got up read our Bibles, prayed, and then just causally wandered around being together. Then, we went out and prayed together for quite a while in the truck. I could tell that the owner was watching me. What I didn't know was that he had been watching me all morning via video camera. Bless his heart, I hope he didn't have it on when I was wearing my old sweats and t-shirt, but he might have!

Through a series of chats, he finally opened up and told me that one of the reasons he sat and watched me is because my registration card said I was a minister. He had learned, the hard way that most ministers can't be trusted. Isn't that a slap in the face? Isn't that a piece of reality pie?

I'm told that some people think of Dallas, Texas, as one of the spiritual capitals of the world. I don't particularly hold that point of view, but a lot of people apparently do. Our motel owner friend confirmed that a lot of ministers were constantly traveling to and from Dallas for seminars, conferences, and conventions of all kinds and often stayed at his motel. But the volume of business was negated by the attitude of these particular customers. He said, "We have not had good experiences with ministers."

With that conversational opener, I had a most interesting talk with him. I found out he had made a Christian commitment years ago, but had drifted away from the Lord. We probably talked for another 45 minutes. When we finished, I felt God saying to me, "I want you to write to those people." So I did. They haven't answered me yet, and I'm asking you to pray for this Oklahoma couple. I believe, deep in my soul, our encounter was the beginning of their day of visitation. I believe God was using me in that situation to be his messenger to them. But, it's their day. They can blow it off. They can say, "We don't want to correspond with that preacher guy. We don't even know him." No. No. No. Be careful. Don't pass up the day of visitation.

Why do I say be careful? Why do I say be quiet and listen for the still, small voice of God? I say it because God is a gentleman, and he comes to us in such loving, gentle ways we can fail to take him seriously. As compared to God, the devil is a slave driver. If you follow him you will end up doing things you never thought you would ever do. I was like that before I came to Christ. I did things that I never thought in my wildest imagination I would ever do. I would find myself in the middle of the biggest mess thinking, "I'm smarter than this. How in the world did I ever get in this mess?" The evil one will drive you like a slave master until you give up on God, others, and yourself.

On the other hand, Jesus, the Good Shepherd will say, "Listen, it would be best if you went this way."

"But I don't want to go that way."

"Are you sure? Come on. Here's the way; walk in it. Come on. Come on."

"I don't want to go that way. I want to do my own thing my own way over here."

"OK."

Then, he'll sadly walk away while we turn up the TV to drown out further communication with him. And being a gentleman, he will let us do it. But he doesn't give up on us even if we turn away and create a new mess for ourselves. He's not a "one strike and your out" God. He is always ready to forgive and forget. That, my friends, is how God, the Holy Spirit, works.

I blew it a week ago. God spoke to me on Thursday and Friday and asked me to go to the hospital in Lafayette and pray with Mrs. Shepler. I felt a little awkward about this because she goes to another church, and I'm not her pastor. As far as I know, she has an excellent pastor. I don't know all the details. What I do know is God had spoken to me about her. Now, I didn't say,

61

"No, I'm not going." I just let myself get busy with my day. You know, busy-busy. Before I was aware, it was 5:00 p.m., and I thought, "Aw, man, you know what Lafayette traffic near Purdue University is going to be like at 5:00. I'm not going to drive over there now."

Well, God spoke to me again early Saturday morning indicating that he still wanted me to go over to pray with and anoint this woman. I knew that for God to speak to me so specifically about praying for someone isn't something that happens every day. So, I should have listened and followed his leading. But I didn't go Saturday as well. On Saturday night, deeply, but gently convicted in my soul, I prayed, "Lord, if you are visiting me about praying for this lady, please give me another opportunity." And I felt God speak to me and say, "Go on Monday." So, on Monday I said to my son, Kevin, "Let's go to Lafayette and pray with Mrs. Shepler." Well, come to find out, Mrs. Shepler had contracted a bad staph infection. She had lost the use of her kidneys and was on dialysis. The doctors were very concerned about her. Not knowing her very well I said, "Mrs. Shepler, may I anoint you and pray for you?"

The Bible says if someone wants prayer and is willing to be anointed, an elder of the church should anoint them. Oil represents the Holy Spirit. There's no power in oil itself, but as you know, there is incredible power in the Holy Spirit. Thus, I asked Mrs. Shepler, "May, I anoint you?" She said yes, and was obviously very happy for the opportunity. And I left the hospital, knowing in my heart of hearts, that God, the gentleman that he is, had visited Mrs. Shepler and me!

Most ministers read their Scriptural text at the beginning of their sermon. I'm going to read mine at the end. Aren't you glad? (I was afraid if I said, "Now in my text," you would think, "Oh, shoot, he's just getting started!")

The story of Moses before the burning bush in Exodus, chapter three, is an awesome example of visitation. It reads:

Moses kept the flock of Jethro, his father-in-law, the priest at Midian. He led the flock to the back side of the desert and came to the mountain of God, even to Horeb. And the angel of the Lord appeared unto him in a flame of fire, out of the midst of a bush. . . . And he looked, and behold, the bush burned with fire, but the bush was not consumed. . . .

Moses was tending sheep. Involved in the everyday responsibilities of earning a living, he noticed that a nearby bush was on fire, something that didn't happen frequently in the desert, but wasn't totally uncommon. It was just a scrawny, old desert bush. Nothing special. It didn't have a steeple on it. It was nothing to worry about, except, the bush was not consumed. Now, that was different!

At this point, Moses had to make a choice. Would he continue with his schedule, his routine, and his responsibilities to his father-in-law's sheep, or would he go and investigate a unique bush? He could have justifiably thought, "That's an interesting bush, but I'm supposed to do some shearing before the sun goes down, and with the price of wool at an all time high, I can't spend the time checking out a bush right now." Moses could have walked away from the bush and missed the most spectacular moment of his life. But, if you choose to read this Exodus chapter three account in your devotions this week, you will find Moses went toward the bush to see what it was, and as a result, God spoke to him from out of the bush and called him to a whole new level of spiritual growth and service. It was his day of visitation.

Now, when your day of visitation comes, it probably won't be a burning bush, so don't look for one. He won't speak to you the same way he did to Moses. He won't speak the same way to you as he speaks to me or any other person. His voice will be unique to you. Yes, there may be some similarities to the experiences of others, but you will recognize the uniqueness of his visitation as you ponder what is happening.

If you'll respond to your day of visitation, God will call your name just as he called Moses by name. You probably won't hear an audible voice, but he will say, "Matt! Lisa! Bryan! Mark!"

And then he will say his own name.

Moses said, "And who are you? And God said, "I Am that I Am is my name."

God's name means he is eternal, sovereign, and always present. Embracing your day of visitation means he is prepared to call your name and save you just as he did Moses and the Children of Israel. He is prepared to lead you out of a life of slavery to sin and dwell with you as you journey to the land he has kept in reserve for you! He is prepared to transform you into a called out, set apart, redeemed, and sanctified child of God. He is prepared to fill you with the Comforter, his Holy Spirit.

Then God said to Moses, "Take off your shoes, for the place you stand is holy ground."

In the shocking, stunning intensity of the moment, Moses was moved to a state of reverence for God. A visitation from God always leads us to a state of reverence for him. In the book of Revelation, it says that when the seventh seal was broken, there was silence in heaven for a half an hour. Heaven, the ultimate place of praise and worship, where the number of angelic choirs cannot be counted, became deathly still by an action of God.

We need days of visitation that move us to reverence. Yes, there's a time to praise and exalt God's presence and goodness. There's a time to sing and shout. There's a time to raise your hands in worship and adoration. In fact, the Scriptures urge us to lift up our hands and praise the Lord. But there's also an awesome, quiet time of reverence, purification, refinement, development, and direction. A time of being so enveloped by a holy hush that nothing seems to matter but your own unworthiness.

It is in the time of reverence that God commissions us and empowers us, just as he did Moses. God commissioned Moses to go to Pharaoh and tell him to let his slave labor, the Children of Israel, leave Egypt. And God promised to provide the power to make this possible.

He said, "Moses, what's that you've got there in your hand?"

Moses said, "A staff."

Oh, an ordinary thing. A staff. Well, Moses always had a staff.

God said, "Throw it on the ground."

Moses threw it on the ground and it became a hissing, wiggling snake. The Scriptures say Moses ran from it.

God said, "Take it by the tail."

Moses did, and the snake became a staff once again.

There's a wonderful promise in this exchange. This passage says, in other words, that God commissions us as we are, as well as the ordinary things of life, to accomplish his purposes. I'm not you and you aren't Tom. Nor are we Dick or Harry. You have your own distinct life, your own personality, and your own distinct skills, talents, and abilities. But, God says, take what you've got and throw it out there and watch him transform it into something powerful and useful. When God gives you a commission, a job to do, he doesn't let you hang out there by yourself. He empowers you to do it. That's the work of the Holy

Spirit.

When I was 21 years old and God confirmed my call to the ministry, I felt intimidated. That's why I'm so intrigued by this passage. I didn't have a bit of seminary training. While I've acquired some biblical education since then, at that time, I had nothing in the way of formal training. But, God had spoken to me. I remember praying, "Lord, I just have my Bible. I've studied it quite a bit, and Mama taught us all the Bible stories. I know something about your word, but that's all I've got." And I felt like God said, "That's all you really need. Throw it out there like the staff of Moses, and I'll empower you." Consequently, there were places I would preach as a very young minister, and men three times my age would come to me and say, "God spoke to me through your message." Isn't it incredible how God takes the "foolish to confound the wise?" He takes the "weak to baffle the strong?" He promises that his power is made perfect in our weakness.

So, in closing, if you haven't heard anything else I said this morning, hear this. Embracing your day of visitation means listening for God's still, small voice. Hear him call your name and then reveal his name unto you. Hear him tell you how he will save you in the manner in which he saves. Let him purify you and move you to a state of reverence. Let him commission you and empower you.

Since I did not read all of Exodus, chapter three, I would ask you to read both chapters three and four this coming week during your devotional time. A lot of what we've talked about this morning will come back to you.

At the risk of redundancy, let me leave you with a final admonition. Don't waste your day of visitation. Resist the temptation a crossroads can bring—the temptation to become angry, bitter, and resentful. Don't shut your eyes, close your ears, stiffen your necks, and harden your hearts. Don't walk away from a burning bush saying, "That thing's too hot. I'm not going near it." Embrace you day of visitation. It may not be an easy day or a very comfortable one, but it will be God's very best for you. Listen for the still, small voice. Let God lead you to a new level, to higher ground!

Chapter 6
Incredible Encounters

In chapter four I talked about how the discovery of leukemia became a day of visitation me. In the fifth chapter I shared a sermon I had preached five months earlier, entitled *Day of Visitation.* As a sequel, I want to share a number of incredible encounters that rounded out this day of visitation. Let me explain. Incredible encounters are those marvelous experiences that unexpectedly occur when your God-directed pathway intersects the God-directed pathway of another person. Psalm 37:23 says, *"A righteous man's steps are ordered of the Lord."* When the steps of two righteous people are ordered of the Lord, and those steps intersect, an incredible encounter begins to take place. And that righteousness does not come from our own goodness. In fact, the Scripture says that our own righteousness is as filthy rags. Nothing we do can earn the grace that God gives us. It is his goodness, his cleansing, and his sacrifice on the cross that makes us righteous. And, as we seek to love him, follow his guidance, and obey his commandments, he promises that he will order our steps. He will also give us incredible encounters.

The First Twenty-four Hours

I could see this verse fulfilled the very first evening of my thirty-one days in the hospital. Beside me for this journey was my wife Pam, my faithful, lifelong companion. I was just starting to realize all of the sacrifices she would make as the result of her commitment and dedication to me. I realized anew that the vows she had made to me years earlier were unconditional as she watched over me constantly and slept on a couch in my room every night.

My hospital room was rather small, the only room available, and I started my 31-day journey by meeting the medical staff members of the sixth floor. I could sense that I was in a special place; every staff person was unusually kind and caring. I have since learned that this sixth floor dedication was a reflection of the entire hospital. Years ago, when I was training for a management position in the Kroger grocery store chain, I was taught that the attitude of the store manager affected everyone else in the store, right down to the young people who bagged the groceries. I've also read that if you pastor a church for 10 years, it will become what you are. That's great motivation for every pastor to become a dedicated servant/leader!

I also sensed that the staff, from top to bottom, was about much more than just doing their job. Yes, they were being paid, but they weren't chasing the dollar. They seemed "called" to their work, and some expressed this very idea in later conversations. Because there was a sense of urgency about my condition, staff members began drawing blood immediately so it could be typed. I desperately needed a transfusion of blood platelets as soon as possible. There was some anxiety in the air since it was unexpectedly difficult to type my blood, and when it was typed, my type was not immediately available. As a result, I waited until 11:00 p.m. for a blood transfusion.

Here again, God was teaching me to lean totally on him. The Scripture says,

"The eternal God is your refuge and underneath are the everlasting arms."

Sometimes, God may put us in situations where the only option is to lean back and put your full weight on his everlasting arms. Thank God for his promises! The proper blood type was found and I began to receive new platelets. The clotting action of the platelets reduced the bleeding from my gums and nose, and I went to sleep, feeling I had entered a dream world.

When I awoke early the next morning, I felt weak from all the stress of the previous day, so I began to meditate and pray. How reassuring to continue to feel the everlasting arms. As a minister, I had spent countless hours telling people how God would be faithful to them in their hour of need. I had stood at many a bedside reading Scripture to the afflicted, praying with them, and assuring them that God would be an ever-present help in time of trouble. How affirming to sense, first-hand, that God was present in my own hour of affliction. I can honestly say that I did not struggle with feelings of fear. I did feel some anxiety about the medical tests I would be given and the new things I would be experiencing, for, as I mentioned earlier, this was my first experience as a hospital patient. My closest encounter with the medical world had been outpatient care for broken bones as the result of minor accidents. This obviously was a stretching experience for me. Stretching experiences help you come to grips with what you really believe. They motivate you to draw from all those things you have preached to other people. How wonderful it is to be on the receiving end of those beliefs and assurances, affirmed that God is all he has claimed to be!

Though I felt weak and faint, I got up out of bed and made my way to the bathroom. As I went in, a song that my niece had sung at a gospel concert a few weeks earlier began going through my mind as though it was being sung to me:

> When my day grows drear,
> Precious Lord, linger near,
> When my life is almost gone;
> Hear my cry,
> Hear my call,
> Hold my hand, lest I fall,
> Take my hand,
> Precious Lord, lead me on.

I cannot describe how vivid and clear that song was to me. It focused me on the Lord's faithfulness. It also reminded me of a time, years earlier, when God had proved his faithfulness to me. In an earlier chapter, I told the story about our son, Allen, being life-lined by helicopter to an Indianapolis hospital after a tragic, near fatal automobile accident. As Pam and I drove south toward Indianapolis, my memory began playing the gospel songs I had sung through the years, all the precious hymns I remembered from childhood. They flowed through my mind one after the other, like an unwinding tape recorder. We read in the Scripture that God will give us a song, yes, a song in the night. Scripture also says that weeping may endure for the night, but joy comes in the morning. During that time of weeping, I found that God would be faithful to everything He had said He would do.

A Doctor Sent by God

My next encounter was with Dr. Schultz, a special physician sent from God. Dr. Schultz is my age. He is married and has four children. An oncologist by training, he is much in demand and a very busy man. As we became acquainted, I realized he was an exceptionally caring person. I've never met a physician who cared for his patients like Dr. Schultz does. I didn't understand this about him at first, but I now realize God was ordering my steps and preparing my way.

Dr. Schultz came into my room and introduced himself. I could see by his facial expressions, his choice of words, and his guarded way of expressing himself that he was very concerned about my condition. He started our first conversation by saying, "We have a tremendous challenge before us." The most recent blood test confirmed I had AML—acute myeloid leukemia—and the level of my leukemia was extremely critical. While I could sense he was trying to be sensitive and considerate, I could also tell that he had reservations about giving me too much hope, because he was so unsure of what the future might be.

71

Though it isn't customary for a patient to pray with their doctor, I had a strong sense that I should pray with Dr. Shultz. So when he finished explaining the various things he was planning to do, I asked if I could pray with him. I'll never forget this moment, for it was a very important moment in my life, and, I believe in his life as well. (This was confirmed several months later when Dr. Schultz told me, "Tom, I believe we were supposed to meet.")

Before I continue telling about my prayer with Dr. Schultz, I want to confess that sometimes, when I had faced adversity in the past, I did not have a good attitude. My thoughts would go in directions they shouldn't go, instead of trusting God. I would question God, and wonder what he was doing. But, I had also learned that when we rebel against the things that afflict us in life, when we resist them with bitterness and anger, and when we refuse to accept our affliction and go into denial, God still loves us. It's a wonderful lesson to learn!

As a young minister, I had the misconception that everything in my life had to be in order before God could use me. Since then, I have realized that God can use me while I'm working through the difficulties of the moment, if I'm willing to submit to his will. He may not use us to the degree we would like, for God is pure, holy, and just and his purposes are perfect. The key to being used of God is an open attitude, a willing heart, and a submissive spirit. When we choose to be willing to accept difficulty and submit to it, God will use us in a powerful way.

At this particular moment with Dr. Schultz, I was able, with God's grace and strength, to be open, ready, willing, and submissive to my affliction. Thus, I believe my stay in the hospital was a day of visitation for both Dr. Schultz and me. I believe God used my time of sickness to teach both of us some important lessons.

I sensed all of this while preparing to pray with Dr. Schultz. I also was very aware of what he had just explained to me—that he would be doing tests and drawing blood for days; that he was going to put me on a machine to lower my blood count; that he was going to surgically put ports in my chest and neck for chemotherapy, other medications, and other medical procedures. He had also told me that in a couple of days, he would begin intense chemotherapy treatment if my white cell count dropped to 50,000. To achieve this number, he was depending on an apheresis machine to extract my blood and remove any cells that were cancerous. These would all be new experiences for me. Without the Lord, they would be very frightening. It's no wonder I felt an urgency to pray with him. But, I believe it was more than praying for my condition. I was praying for this special man. So I asked him, "Dr. Schultz, I have a strange request. Would you mind if I had prayer with you?"

"Sure," he said, and he sat down on the bed.

He, Pam, and I joined hands. What a wonderful privilege! I began to pray as well as cry. A holy awe settled down on the room. I remember praying, "Lord, I'm putting my life in this man's hands. I've preached on submission all of my life. I'm going to submit to him. I'm going to do whatever he tells me to do. I'm asking you to give him guidance, to give him wisdom, and to give him insight into my disease. I'm asking for your hand to be upon him. Obviously, I trust him, but I recognize that he is human and you are the great physician. Guide his mind. Guide his hands. Be close to him and help us through this experience. In Jesus' name, Amen."

I can't adequately explain how I felt at the end of my prayer, but I know a personal connection was forged in prayer that only the power of the Holy Spirit makes possible. I've deeply loved Dr. Schultz ever since that moment. I believe he feels the same way toward me. Prayer bonds people together. Life-long relationships can develop through prayer that won't happen any other way.

What an incredible encounter with Dr. Schultz! Little did I know of the friendship that would develop and the good times we would spend together. I keep a picture in my office of Dr. Schultz and me with our arms around each other. Under the picture it reads:

I thank my God at every remembrance of you. (Philippians 1:3)

In the next few hours the medical staff checked my heart (chemotherapy is very hard on the heart) and put ports in my neck so I could be connected to the apheresis machine. As I understand it, the machine extracts blood through one of the ports, spins it at a high rate of speed to extract the white blood cells, and then returns it to the body through the second port. With my white cell count at 137,000, most of the extracted cells were classified as "trashed cells," and it was important to lower their volume to 50,000 in order for chemotherapy to be effective. My blood was like sludge. They showed me a vial of it after it had settled for a few moments, and I could see that it had a granular, charcoal-looking substance in it. It's still amazing to me that I didn't suffer a brain hemorrhage or some kind of a stroke. God was very gracious to me, for which I am very, very thankful.

God Prepared an Angel

With the goal of lowering my white count to 50,000, Dr. Schultz was hopeful of beginning chemotherapy on Thursday, Thanksgiving Day. I was taken to a surgical unit where surgeons and nurses were to put the ports in my neck. And in this group was a very special nurse who God had prepared as an angel for me.

I saw these small miracles happen again and again. I cannot sufficiently emphasize in this little book how faithful God is regarding all of the details of life. He knew I was anxious. He knew I had never experienced a surgical procedure before. And now they were getting ready to cut into an artery in my neck, just to the right and below my chin. I needed assurance.

I remember lying there listening to the nurses visit with each other while they were doing various things in and out of the room. One of them was talking about her horses. So, I piped up, "We have horses," trying to get my mind on something other than a knife piercing my neck artery. "We have riding horses we use for recreation and vacations. My wife and I often go camping and take a couple of riding horses with us." Not thinking of anything else to say, I stopped talking and tried to relax while the ports were put in my neck. As they began to sterilize the skin, and make the cuts, I asked the Lord to send me an angel, for this was the first moment since we had come to the hospital that Pam was not at my side. I needed assurance.

After the surgical procedure was under way, a nurse came bedside, put both elbows on the bedrail and began to pat me on the left shoulder. She said, "So, you have horses. What kind of horses do you have?"

I said, "Quarter horses."

She said, "Do you ever go camping?"

"Yes. We recently went to the Winamac state park to ride and early in October we camped in Brown County."

She said, "We just went to Brown County with our horses."

A conversation began to develop. Even now, tears come to my eyes as I realize that the eternal God, creator of heaven and earth, would be so sensitive to the needs of an anxious and hurting man that he would send a nurse to converse with him about something familiar to him. I believe God nudged that nurse to be my assuring angel in that moment of anxiety.

The surgical procedure was successful and I was connected to the apheresis machine. I had only been on the machine for about ninety minutes when I began to feel a change in my head. I asked the nurse who was monitoring the procedure if it was common for people to feel things while they were on this machine. She expressed alarm and asked what I was feeling. I told her I didn't think there was need to be concerned, for I was beginning to feel a relief of pressure in my head. Later I learned that my high white count had caused feelings of pressure in my head, something with which I had learned to live. What a blessing to feel the relief from pressure!

How special to be in the midst of small miracles by the dozen! How wonderful that God would give someone the wisdom to create a machine that takes blood out of your body, spins it, removes the harmful content, and then puts it back in! I realized anew that the Savior just keeps performing miracles. Sometimes He will just touch you, or let you touch him. Other times he will use a process, or a man-made machine. Since we are surrounded by miracles we often overlook, we should constantly pray, "God, please forgive us for when we take you and your acts of kindness for granted."

The next morning I was returned to surgery for the insertion of a Hickman port in my chest. The port contains two rubber tubes that allow one to receive medications very quickly and be transfused at any time. Little did I know that during the next few months endless medications would be given to me.

God Sent an Insight

While waiting anxiously to be taken to surgery, Tony Winters

76

walked into my room. Tony pastors a neighboring church in our area and is highly respected minister in our community. I didn't know Tony well, and we had never developed anything more that a casual friendship, though we had shared funeral officiating responsibilities. Indianapolis is two hours away from our community, so I was more than surprised to see him. What surprised me even more was the manner in which he came into my room. In past encounters, Tony, at least toward me, had always seemed somewhat mild-mannered. He was never forward or the slightest bit aggressive. He always approached me in a soft tone of voice. But, as he came bedside with a small bottle of anointing oil, his manner was more forward and focused, as though he was on a mission of some kind.

As he spoke to me, I realized that this was the case. In his South African accent he said, "Tom, God sent me here today. When I got up this morning, God spoke to me and said, 'Go to Indianapolis, and tell Tom Robbins I'm not finished with him yet.' Now I know they're waiting for you in surgery, but I must pray for you." And he began to pray, while opening the bottle of oil and anointing me. Tony prayed a gentle but powerful prayer, asking God to touch me, to help me with the immediate surgery, to take me through this time of crisis safely, and to raise me up for further ministry.

Please remember that I had been given the verses from II Kings about extended life. I had also received numerous impressions from God that he was going to take care of me. Even so, I needed assurance at that moment. Isn't it amazing how God supplies all of our needs? I have absolutely no question in my mind that God sent Tony to minister to me, and I'll always be grateful for his obedience to God.

I need to add here how important it is for each of us to be obedient to God's voice. I can't help but wonder how many times I've passed up important opportunities to minister in his name because I wasn't in tune with Him. It's so important to start the day with God, to take time for his word and for prayer. I'm sure it was in an early morning hour when God spoke to Tony, and being in tune with the Lord, he was obedient. What an impact his obedience had on me!

I went on to surgery and had the Hickman inserted in my chest. It was an adjustment to come back to my room with these two tubes coming from the area of my heart. Later that day, glad to see my brother with whom I always joked, and showing him my tubes, I said with a smile, "Well Jim, Jesus and I have leukemia." He looked at me and broke out laughing until he realized that this time I wasn't joking. He replied, "Tom, that says it all, doesn't it? You and Jesus have leukemia."

I deeply meant that statement. I knew Jesus would never leave me or forsake me. He said he would always be with us. So it was safe to conclude, if I was going through a valley, he would be going with me. When we are connected to Jesus, he shares our sorrows, our afflictions, our difficulties, and sends his Holy Spirit to comfort us. Live or die, everything was going to be all right.

God Sent Additional Assurance

Mornings in a hospital can be quite delightful. I would often awaken while it was still dark and pray. Or I would turn on a little light I had on my bed and read from the Book of Psalms. I enjoy the Psalms. They speak of so many different experiences, and much strength can be drawn from these wonderful prayers and poems.

Occasionally, I would listen to the tape player I kept beside my bed. One of my favorite tapes was one our son, Scott, had made of encouraging songs. On the morning following my port surgery I began listening to this tape when Ray Boltz's song,

Thank You for Giving to the Lord began to play. Through this song the Lord gave me another incredible encounter

As I was listening the song came to the phrase, "I turned and saw this young man, and he was smiling as he came," I saw something out of the corner of my eye, and when I turned to look, I saw an image of Tony Bench, the nephew of Cincinnati Reds baseball legend Johnny Bench, in the corner of the room.

One of the things I believe God does sometimes during a day of visitation is answer the prayers that have been on your heart for a long time. Several years earlier, Tony found himself in our local jail. The star of a rock band, he had been arrested after a party, where he had been entertaining. While in jail, he began reading the Bible. After his release, the jail chaplain suggested that he attend church, so Tony chose to visit our church. I remember sitting on the platform seeing this young man, his wife, and their two small children, though I didn't have any idea who they were. Throughout the service I felt God was saying to me, "Look at that man. Notice that man." God made him stand out to me.

Because of those feelings, I went to Tony after the service and asked him who he was. He told me his story, including being released from jail. Wanting to know him better I invited him to meet me later in the week for coffee. That first meeting led to several coffees and lunches, and before you know it, Tony and his wife were attending services regularly. I was thrilled when he opened his heart to the Lord. Tony was one of the best singers I had ever heard (I could understand why he was a star in a rock band), and he began singing in the church, as well as singing with me. We performed a lot of music together.

But, this story does not end well. During the following year, Tony got mixed up in a messy situation, left his wife, went back to Oklahoma where his mother lived, and resumed his drinking.

He called me two or three times while intoxicated, to tell me how sorry he was and what a mess he had made of his life. We lost touch and I heard nothing more until word came that Tony had been killed in an automobile accident. I had a major heartache over Tony Bench.

Since that time, I had been haunted with the question of what happened to Tony. Was he in heaven? Did he really connect with the Lord in the first place? Did he reconnect with the Lord before he was killed? What caused him to do some of the things he did? God knew I had many questions in my heart about Tony and his eternal destiny. How awesome that, during this time of cancer, my day of visitation, God let me see an image of Tony Bench in the corner of my room while listening to a song about heaven. To this day I don't know if I had a vision or I saw an angel posing as Tony. All I know is that my mind was miles away from thinking of Tony Bench when an incredible encounter took place, and I saw what I saw!

But, that was only the first of two wonderful encounters. The second one happened that same day when one of Dr. Schultz's team physicians came into my room and introduced himself. Dr. Fraiz immediately reminded me of my nephew, Dan Robbins, in his looks and mannerisms. Both men are very special people! When he saw the Bible laying on the table next to my bed, he asked where I was reading. That warm introduction birthed many conversations. Dr. Fraiz became a very special Christian brother. We prayed together, cried together, and shared together. I'll always be grateful for him and his Christian fellowship.

God Showed Me His Blessings

During that first week in the hospital, God laid it on my heart to create a new "Blessings Book." Since Allen's (our third son) accident I had been journaling the blessings, miracles, and special

80

things God was doing in our lives. Believing with my whole heart that God can "work all things for good," I began writing down those good things. You may recall, from a previous chapter, the financial help we received during Allen's hospital stay. That financial help was recorded in my Blessings Book. Some blessings were large and some were small. God's hand was in each one.

The word "book" is a bit misleading, since what I did was glue together some legal pads on which I could scribble down the blessings soon after they happened. My first book contained 37 pages of blessings. Each line of every page recorded something God had done. You would be amazed at some of the things recorded there. They will remind you of an old gospel song I grew up singing:

Count your blessings; name them one by one . . .
And it will surprise you what the Lord has done.

How easy it is to forget God goodness and slip into an attitude of, "What have you done for me lately?" A Blessing Book is a wonderful antidote for that kind of diseased thinking. Some of the lines in my first book read as follows:

"Our good friends gave us half a beef to help us with groceries through the winter."

"God saved my son's life."

"My car quit on the way back from visiting a hospital in Fort Wayne. I prayed beside the road, it started, and I was able to drive home."

Regardless of the size of the incident, or the degree of importance that it may have to others, I would try and record what I thought were the special things God was doing in our lives. Now, I felt impressed to start a new Blessings Book. So I acquired a fresh legal pad and wrote on the top of the first page,

"BLESSINGS FROM MY LEUKEMIA EXPERIENCE" and the date. This was followed by a series of blessing lines: Meeting Dr. Schultz; Tony Winters visit; Meeting Dr. Fraiz; Seeing Tony Bench; A visit from my brother Jim, etc.

That afternoon, as Dr. Schultz made his rounds, he noticed my legal pad, with its scribbly writing, and asked, "What are you doing? Writing a letter to your parish?"

I said, "No. That's my Blessings Book."

He said, "What?"

I said, "That's my Blessings Book. I believe God is going to bring blessings through this cancer experience. In fact, he already has, and I'm writing them down." He looked at me, very stunned, and muttered, "I wish more people would do that." I don't share this anecdote to compliment myself; counting one's blessings is what Christians do! However, Dr. Schultz's response reminded me how foreign this practice might be to those who don't understand that when we walk with the Lord, all things *do* work together for good. Again, this was an encounter that ministered to both of us.

God Granted a Long Standing Request

Of all the experiences I have had over the years, I would probably rate this next encounter as close to the top of the list. My encounter began on Wednesday, the day before Thanksgiving, with a group of St. Vincent nurses called chemo nurses. As we became acquainted, I learned that many of them felt called in some very personal way to work with cancer patients. I say "called" because some were Christians, but others had experienced cancer themselves, or had been closely involved with a loved one who died from cancer. Isn't it interesting how God uses our difficult experiences to put us where we need to be?

This particular morning a chemo nurse, by the name of Susie, came to my room and introduced herself, saying she would be my nurse. I could immediately tell she was a Christian. She had heard that I was a minister, and as we got to know each other, I shared some of my anxieties with her. The next morning she came into my room and very brightly said, "God spoke to me and gave me a scripture verse for you, Zephaniah 3:17:

For your God is with you.
He is mighty to save.
He will take great delight in you.
He will quiet you with His love.
He will rejoice over you with singing.

I was surprised that she would be quoting from Zephaniah. A lot of Christians would have trouble finding the book of Zephaniah in the Bible let alone be reading from it! But, I was awestruck by her quote. You may recall that at my first anointing in the church on November 20, I had three requests. The least important was that God would touch me physically, if he so desired. The second was that He would help me with my fears— dissolve my fears. The first, and most important, was that I would suffer honorably. I wanted to always possess the Spirit of Christ. I wanted to be pleasing to the Lord. I didn't want to disappoint those who looked up to me for spiritual leadership.

God reminded me of those requests the minute Susie quoted verse seventeen. God, speaking through the prophet Zephaniah, and Susie, his chemo nurse messenger, was saying he would take great delight in me and quiet me with His love. Most importantly, he was going to rejoice over me.

Susie had no knowledge of my November 20 prayer circle of friends, or my three requests. But, God knew, and he gave her that verse for me! I began to cry. When I finally collected myself, I told her, "You need to know why the verse you quoted is so important to me. God used you to answer my prayer by giving me this promise." Then I told her about my three requests. But, that's not the end of the story.

There is a family in our church by the name of Troyer whom I love very much. I have had a number of occasions to minister to this family since they have suffered more than their share of grief. I spent many hours with Mrs. Troyer as she battled cancer and then officiated at her funeral. The grandmother of the Troyer family, Elizabeth Waits, passed away, and I officiated at her funeral the week before I discovered I had leukemia. Other family members struggled with one crisis after another. Through all of these difficulties, I observed how much these family members cared for one another, how they upheld and supported one another through thick and thin. It was remarkable. I even mentioned from the pulpit that if I was ever sick, I would like for one of the Troyers to take care of me. And, sure enough, when I was hospitalized, one of the family members, Randy, called and asked, "Is there something we can do? You've often said you wanted the Troyers to look after you."

When you are in chemotherapy, visitors are often restricted. This was the case with me. My immunity was so low that visitors were not allowed in the room, and family members had to wear gowns and masks. So, Troyer family members were not allowed to even visit me. But, the Lord gave me special care anyway. Apparently, he hears our requests as well as the comments we make from the pulpit, for I soon discovered that Susie, the Christian chemo nurse was—you guessed it—a Troyer! I couldn't believe it. I was floored! God doesn't miss a single detail. He just continued to prove that he is "able to give exceedingly and abundantly above all we can we ask or think." Thank God for Susie Troyer.

The following day was Thanksgiving Day. It was time to start my chemotherapy and it was intimidating. Due to the extreme dosage of chemotherapy I had to take, and the intensity of the poison I was to be given, the chemo nurses had to wear gowns, masks, and gloves. It is frightening when the medical caretakers come into the room, protecting every inch of their skin, from the poison they're going to inject through your Hickman port directly into your heart and body.

Needless to say, I was dealing with some anxiety, asking the Lord to help me. Having seen so many suffer from chemotherapy, I've had nightmares about what chemotherapy is like. Guess who the administering nurse was Thursday morning for chemotherapy? You guessed it—Susie Troyer! She sat by my bed in gown, mask, and gloves, hooked up the hoses and said, "I'm going to pray with you." What an absolutely tremendous experience, to have a nurse, God's messenger, pray with you before your chemotherapy. How faithful our God is!

Some may ask, if God gives a promise to touch you, why do you need medical treatment? I, too, had that question go through my own mind. And, it's interesting to note how God always knows the thoughts and the questions that may come to your mind. For example, God had clearly given me the promise of II Kings 20:5: "I have heard your prayer and seen your tears, and I will heal you, and I will add 15 years to your life." However, it's important to keep reading. Verse seven says, "Then Isaiah said, 'Prepare a poultice of figs,' and they did so and applied it to the boil, and he recovered." Yes the promise was a healing touch and an extension of life, but the means to wholeness was a medicating poultice. I had prayed with Dr. Schultz and submitted myself to his wisdom and care. Chemotherapy is what he prescribed. Thus, I was confident that God was guiding in every detail, for he had promised that if we acknowledge the Lord in all of our ways, he directs our path.

85

God Sends Encouragement

Thanksgiving Day was exceptional for many reasons. Even though it was the first day of what was to become a grueling chemotherapy regimen, the scripture Susie had given me the day before was ringing in my ears. What a special promise!

It was also the day I received word that my two assistant pastors, Chris Edgington and Howard France, had called the church together the evening before for intercessory prayer on my behalf. Approximately 150 people assembled to pray, and my prayer partner, Bryan Jaberg, was anointed on my behalf. Family by family they came forward to the altar to pray for me. What could be more encouraging and supportive than to have the people to whom you have ministered reciprocate on your behalf? They will never know how much this meant to me.

Rev. Terri White, who pastors a church in near-by Twelve Mile, Indiana, attended the prayer service and sent me a note about it:

Dear Tom,

I want to share with you that I went to an incredible service Wednesday evening. A couple of people had called me to let me know about the service, and I called [and notified] our prayer chains. I came home mid-afternoon and lay down on the couch for just a second, but went to sleep. When my eyes opened it was dark outside. My husband was home and I said, "What time is it?" He replied, "6:35."

I flew off the couch, jumped in the car, and made it to your church in record time. And I was so very glad I did. I must be honest. I wept through the entire service. I sat back and watched a group of dedicated, concerned, hurting people, who were lifting not just their pastor, but their very dear friend

86

up in prayer. I was so overwhelmed with the essence of love that permeated the sanctuary.

If you have ever doubted if the Lord has used you to do His work and spread His Word, let my small witness confirm that He has chosen you. I watched as people came forward one by one, family by family, to lay hands on your behalf. I listened as they read the scripture that you've been praying, II Kings 20, and found myself wanting to have a pen so I could write it on the palm of my hand so I didn't forget it. What a perfect [scriptural] passage and testimony to your faith.

In the past several weeks, I've kept searching for a connecting thought for the holidays for my church. The one line that keeps coming back is this: Will you be home for the holidays? As I try to convey to the congregation, being home for the holidays isn't about an address, cooking a big meal, or the gifts you put under the Christmas tree. Home is about where your heart is. I spoke of being at Skinner Chapel on that special Wednesday, and I told them that you said you've never felt closer to Jesus, and I read 2 Kings 20. What became such a reality to me is that no matter where you and Pam are this Christmas, whether you're in the hospital, at home, or wherever, your family will indeed be home for the holidays with Jesus. What a blessing! What a praise!

You're being prayed for every day by so many people—ones that love you and ones that have never met you. I am humbled by your strength and faith in this incredibly difficult time, but yet I know that every minute will be used as a testimony to the power of the Lord and His commitment to His children. I pray that you will feel His presence everyplace you go and everything you go through. May you feel him snuggle beside you, holding your hand, arms around you, whispering in your ear how much he loves you.

If you need anything, please don't hesitate to let me know.

Love in Christ,

Terri

Wow! A letter delivered from the Lord Himself wouldn't have meant any more to me because it was, in fact, a letter from the Lord delivered by Terri. I'll always be indebted to her for that note of encouragement.

I also received a note from my brother-in-law, Jesse Stout. Jesse has ministered to me many times throughout my life. His note was entitled, *Reflections in the Early Morning*. Jesse, too, has found that early morning times with God help makes life worth living. He writes:

Tom,

I believe several people have told you that while they were reading and meditating, God assured them your work here is not done. I believe you have felt a similar assurance. As I was heading for Vietnam, I felt directed to Psalm 91:7, "A thousand may fall at your side, and ten thousand at your right hand, but it will not come near to you." This verse did not keep me from feeling threatened, being injured, and sometimes feeling very scared. But God did keep his affirmation to me.

I write this to assure you that when God speaks, he

has taken everything into account and is able to deliver us. You may have things happen, like yesterday's difficulty in breathing that will alarm you. These things are often allowed to keep us trusting God, and to verify, once again, that by Him we live, move, and have our being. Rest in the goodness of God and what He has told your heart.

Your loving brother,

Jesse

What a wonderful letter of encouragement from one who earned a purple heart for his courageous service in the Vietnam War! In his note, Jesse referred to breathing difficulties. I neglected to mention that, while the Hickman port was being inserted into my chest, the surgeon nicked my lung, and my lung collapsed. I had great difficulty breathing for several minutes. It was a somewhat anxious moment!

God Sent My Sons

The highlight of the day was a visit from our four sons. While Tom, his wife Trisha, and their little boy, Braxten, live near Peru, Scott, Allen, and Kevin were attending a Bible school in Dallas, Texas. With the financial help of some friends, they were able to fly home and join Pam and me at the hospital for a Thanksgiving Day family reunion. Since my immune system was compromised by chemotherapy, the boys needed to be gowned and wear masks as they approached my bedside. I was touched by their willingness to spend the entire day inside, even though it is so uncomfortable to be masked the whole time.

Tom suggested that they all pray for me. I can still visualize this special moment as they joined hands with their mother around my bed and Tom led off. It is a Christian father's dream fulfilled to hear his children talk intimately with God, especially when their petitions are on your behalf. Prior to their prayer, Kevin and Scott both shared scripture verses God had given them. Kevin's scripture was John 11, "Now a man named Lazarus was sick. He was from Bethany, the city of Mary and her sister, Martha. So they came to Jesus and said, 'Lord, the one you love is sick.' And when He heard this, Jesus said, 'This sickness will not end in death. No. It is for God's glory so that God's son may be glorified through it.'" I was affirmed, again, that Kevin passage contained the same promise that had been given to others though he didn't know about those other passages.

Scott handed me a piece of paper on which he had hand copied Psalm 103. I was so touched that I later memorized this entire Psalm while in the hospital:

> *Praise the Lord, O my soul;*
> *all my inmost being, praise His holy name.*
> *Praise the Lord, O my soul,*
> *and forget not all His benefits—*
> *who forgives all your sins*
> *and heals all your diseases,*
> *who redeems your life from the pit*
> *and crowns you with love and compassion,*
> *who satisfies your desires with good things*
> *so that your youth is renewed like the eagle's.*

What an incredible encouragement at a time of sickness!

Later that day, my two older sons, Tom and Scott, each gave me a handwritten note much too personal to be shared in this book. I mention these acts of kindness because I had often struggled with feelings of failure as a father. I was busy—too busy—as the boys were growing up. Consumed with the challenges of pastoring, I wasn't as available to them as I should have been. But in this special day of visitation, these notes from my sons, told me that God had been faithful despite my deficiencies. God had provided for them, despite my failures. In these notes, they expressed their love and admiration in a way that was extremely humbling. This may seem like a strong statement, but I've often said that those notes were worth my leukemia experience. I wrote in my Blessings Book, "There were four prayers that were worth it all, and two notes that touched my deepest self."

If I couldn't be home with the family on Thanksgiving Day, being with family in a hospital room was the next best thing! And Pam did an amazing job of making my room as cozy and homey as possible. She covered the walls with pictures and two bulletin boards containing snapshots of our family, friends, horses, and motorcycle rides. My favorite pictures were on my table right next to my bed—a picture of Braxten, my grandson, and a picture of our four sons and daughter-in-law with Pam and me. How encouraging it was to wake up and see my loved ones. My heart goes out to people who don't have family and friends in their hour of need.

My sister-in-law, Kathy, created a poster of II Kings 20:1-6 (large print) and place it on the wall directly in front of me. Every time I looked straight ahead I saw God's promise to me: *I will heal you. I have seen your tears, and I will add 15 years to your life. I have heard your prayer.* How awesome to gaze again and again at this special message from the Lord.

I marvel how God, at our lowest point, provides the encouragement we need in many ways and forms, and through many people. My encouragement came from medical staff, my congregation, fellow ministers, relatives, and my immediate family. In fact the visit from my oldest sister, Sharon, was one of the greatest blessings. Sharon lives in Las Vegas. When she heard I had leukemia, she took a week off work and flew to

Indianapolis to be with me. I was touched by her decision. Since Sharon is a dozen years older than I, she had left home as I was growing up and I never spent that much time with her.

I heard a knock on my hospital room door. As the door opened, I heard the Lord whisper, "I'm sending you your mother." Sharon came in the room, approached the bed, leaned down and kissed me on the cheek, and said, "I'm coming in mother's place."

Unbelievable! The mother I was so close to, and who died in my arms, paid me a visit in the form of my older sister! God obviously revealed the special nature of this visit to both Sharon and me at the same time. What an incredible encounter!

Chapter 7

"Let not your heart be troubled . . .
I will send the Comforter"

The Gospel of John, chapter 14, has always been a favorite of mine. Jesus begins by saying, "Let not your heart be troubled." He then speaks of leaving this earth and returning to his Father. We know from the larger biblical context of this chapter that these comments of Jesus created distress for his disciples. They had great difficulty comprehending what he was saying, and what the implications might be. Knowing this, Jesus made them a promise: "I'm going to send you the Comforter, the Holy Spirit." This is the same Holy Spirit who is with us today, and his primary ministry is one of comfort.

While I experienced many blessings during my time in the hospital, there also were numerous moments of pain, anxiety, and despair. It was a "walk through the valley of the shadow of death" time in my life, a time of review, a time for a lot of "what if" questions, and a time of wondering about the future. At first, medically speaking, my prognosis was not optimistic. Though God had given me promises based on scripture, which I was holding onto very tightly, I found myself processing a multitude of questions. Was God going to heal me immediately? Was the treatment regimen going to be long, painful, and debilitating? What if God decided, for some reason, to withhold his touch? Had I completed everything I was created to accomplish in life? Was I the minister/servant God wanted me to be? Did I truly serve the people he wanted me to serve? Did I proclaim and teach his word the way I should? These, and many more questions like them came at me from all directions.

Well, the Lord knows our thoughts, including our questions. And he sends the Comforter to us in many ways. One of those ways is the affirmation and encouragement of other people. So, as I wrestled with questions of what had been accomplished, and whether I had really been faithful to God's word as a pastor, I began to receive dozens of notes and letters. Though some were very personal and contain compliments of which I am not worthy, I think it is important to share some of them with you, and show how the Comforter graciously focuses God's affirmation and encouragement on one's troubling moments of question and doubt. Given the limitations of space, I have chosen just a handful, in paraphrased form, as examples.

Haley Hostetler, a new Christian in our church, wrote:

> *I believe that you are a messenger from God. You probably are needed in heaven, but on earth there are so many who need to hear the word that will help them open their eyes. You have that gift. We pray each morning and night that God will let you stay here and continue to bring more people to him.*

Mike Wolf wrote:

> *Because of your wonderful way of communicating God's word to me, I know beyond a shadow of a doubt that the most important thing I can do in this life is serve the Lord—to walk with him, to love Him, to do his will.*

Mike and Jan Baker wrote:

> *You have a gift. A gift to bring people back to God. A gift that will not be lost. Our prayers, our hopes, and our love are with you.*

Nick and Autum Salsbury are a young couple in our church with a brand new family. They recently made a commitment to Christ. I clearly remember officiating at their wedding three years ago. They wrote:

We want to let you know how much you mean to us. You have been with us during two of the best times of our lives. It was an honor to have you marry us and baptize us. In the last year you have taught us more about God and how to be good Christians than anyone in our lives. Your messages are truly sent from God. We continue to learn. You have touched our lives so deeply that they will be forever changed for the better. Tom, we really admire you and respect you and your family. We want to thank you so much for all you have done in our lives. If there is anything you or your family needs, please let us know. You are in our hearts and our prayers.

The way Rick Kellam writes, he could be a preacher himself!

Dear Tom,

I have admired you for as long as I can remember. Initially, I was drawn to your cool cars and bikes and your quick-witted sense of humor. But I am most impressed by your unwavering, deep, spiritual commitment and leadership.

Like a true leader, you have given support and counsel in challenging situations.

Now, facing great personal adversity, you have an opportunity to stand tall, meet the challenge, and walk through the fire as you have taught others to do.

According to the account in the third chapter of Daniel, King Nebuchadnezzar couldn't believe his

95

*eyes when he looked into the furnace and saw four
people walking in the midst of the fire, since he had
only cast in three. When three were put to the
ultimate test, one more was present: "... and the form
of the fourth is like the Son of God."*

*If King Nebuchadnezzar were here to observe your
situation, he would be astonished, just as he was
then. He would see what we all see—Tom Robbins,
in the midst of the fire, facing the ultimate test, yet
walking amidst the fire with another form right
beside him, the Son of God.*

*You continue to be in my thoughts and prayers.
Thank you for your inspiration.*

How can you put a value on letters like these? It was like the
Comforter had inserted a port directly into my soul and was
pumping me full of spiritual antidotes—affirmation and
encouragement—to counteract the poison of anxiety, doubt, and
despair. Ah, the blessed, comforting work of the Holy Spirit.
God was blessing me with comfort therapy as well as
chemotherapy!

Kim Fouts had been the girl next door. During the 21 years
we lived near Mexico, Indiana, we were the next-door neighbors
of the Fouts family. Kim was one of two children who grew up
with our four sons. Since it was a time of extreme busyness
(which I've mentioned previously), I don't remember much about
Kim other than greeting her and occasionally teasing her as she
played in the backyard with our boys. To my shame, I don't
remember having any meaningful conversations with her. I
always tried to be kind to her, and I remember a few times when
she seemed sad, I would ask her if she was okay.

I share this background with Kim's letter, for it illustrates how closely others watch and observe us even though we may be totally unaware of what is going on in their hearts. It also illustrates the way a few "seeds of kindness"—inadvertent gestures of recognition or concern—can produce tremendous results. The Bible says that the kingdom of heaven is like a mustard seed. Though it is the smallest of seeds, when planted, it becomes a tree that fills the whole earth. What an interesting statement—fills the whole earth. What it is saying is that small can be both beautiful and powerful!

I realized, again, the power of this truth when I received Kim Byrum's (the former Kim Fouts) letter:

Tom,

You were like a father to me when I was young. You were there for me when my marriage fell apart, and I was ashamed to be alive. You were there for me when my mother passed away. Your life has made such a huge difference to me. A seed was planted in me when I was young, a seed that has blossomed and influenced both my husband and step-children, all of whom know the Lord. You and your family will always have a special place in my heart. I don't understand why God is letting you go through this trial, but that is not for us to understand. We all must trust and keep our faith that God has a plan. I love you and your family, and I will have you in my thoughts and prayers.

Several months ago I was riding my palomino horse down our country road, just enjoying the evening. As I rode past the Grays' home, the first house east of us, I noticed that their little grandson, Lukey, was out in the yard. I could tell that the horse fascinated him, so I stopped, said hi, and got off the horse. Mr.

97

Gray, his grandfather, came out and began looking at the horse as well. Sensing Lukey wanted to come closer, I asked if he wanted to pet the horse and led the horse over to him so he could pet it on the nose. He was delighted, so I asked if he wanted to sit on the horse and go for a ride, if it was OK with Grandpa. Grandpa nodded yes, and I set Lukey up on the horse and walked him around for several minutes. Wanting to continue my ride, I lifted Lukey off the horse, remounted, said Goodbye, and went on my way.

Frankly, I had forgotten about that event. But in the notes and letters that kept coming, I received a note from the Grays. They said that Lukey was praying for me, and for my leukemia. He had told his kindergarten class about it, and every day, at lunchtime, they prayed for me. My heart was deeply touched, for I believe children play a very important role in the kingdom of God. In Scripture it says, *"A little child shall lead them."* I've often wondered if the simple faith of children doesn't have far more impact on situations than we realize? I'll always be grateful for the prayers of Lukey and his kindergarten friends. Since then I've seen Lukey many times and thanked him for praying for me. He's always excited to see me. Isn't it amazing how a special bond across generational lines began with a few moments on the back of a horse? Nothing was said about God. Nothing was said about church. Nothing was said about Christianity. Lukey just rode my horse. Once again, I realized the value of seeds of kindness, and how God can use those powerful seeds for his glory!

I also want to share a neat note I received from a little girl in our church named Missy. Sometimes when you're really sick, you just need a chuckle. It reads:

Dear Pastor Tom,

I hope your cold is feeling
better so you can have a Happy
Christmas!

Love Missy

I could only wish that what I had was a cold!

I received other notes that contained specific lines God used to comfort me. Dan Elkins, a good friend, wrote at the bottom of a card:

I wish I could take the bullet for you on this one. You know what I mean. God Bless!

It's so comforting to have a member of the body of Christ make a statement of that magnitude: " I wish I could take the bullet for you." Scripture says *"No greater love has any man than this, that he lay down his life for his friends."* This is what Jesus did out of his love for us. When God's love is in our heart, it's incredible how unselfish we can become. I saw Dan's heart in his "right to the point" statement.

After two weeks, the chemotherapy regimen was wearing me down to a frazzle, but the notes and letters just kept coming. One card was signed with 20 or 25 signatures. It came from the varsity basketball team our son Tom coaches. They not only signed this wonderful card of encouragement, they enclosed forty dollars in cash! The team had spontaneously taken a collection among themselves to help with food and other incidentals at the hospital. What a remarkable thing for a group of teenagers to do!

To me, the most amazing thing about the comforting ministry of the Holy Spirit was the way in which he laid my travail, both physical and spiritual, on people's hearts. I can't explain this very well, but I sometimes sensed there was more going on than just assurance and encouragement regarding my physical distress. I even wondered if Satan was out to destroy our ministry. What I can say is that the Comforter burdened the heart of people I hardly knew in sacrificial ways.

A young man named Zack showed up in my hospital room. I had met Zack and chatted briefly with him a few times, but I didn't know him very well. Nevertheless, he began our visit by telling me how extremely burdened he became when he heard I had leukemia. He went on to say that for three days, he had been fasting and praying for me! For a casual acquaintance to have that level of prayer burden for me was unbelievable! Here, again, the Holy Spirit, the Comforter, was engaging others in this massive struggle.

My sister Miriam, who faithfully stood by me during my sickness, has a good friend named Jan, a women I've met but hardly know. According to Miriam, Jan was "praying with tears" for me. She was following my updates on the internet (one of the assistant pastors was posting updates of my situation on our church website). Jan would check the internet and then worship, sing, and pray, devoting several moments of intercessory prayer on my behalf. Amazing!

A friend of Paul and Irma Moshesh, whom I had never met, stopped by the hospital to tell me he heard about my sickness by cell phone while he was sitting in his car. He said, while crying, that he felt God was telling him to pray for me.

Encouragement came from many directions and many people, for God knew I was vulnerable to anxiety, doubt, and despair. I've often said that I'm hard proof God can use the weak and unlikely for his eternal purposes. I also want to reiterate my discomfort with some of these notes and letters. God knows I am not worthy of any praise or recognition for trying to serve the Lord. God must be given the glory for any goodness that has come through my life and ministry. I share them as a thank offering for the work of the Comforter. And, I encourage you to embrace the comforting work of the Holy Spirit. The God of comfort knows exactly what you need, and he will be there to affirm and encourage you in your darkest hour.

Let me finish this chapter with one more anecdote, one that gave me another infusion of hope, as well as a glimpse of what my future might still hold. For fifteen years I had been befriending Bill Holler, the owner of a motorcycle shop near our home. The first time I stopped by for some service on my motorcycle, it was with a sense of divine appointment. Bill was a man with a lot of problems. He lived a rough lifestyle and was very far from the Lord. Through a series of "shoptalk" conversations, we became acquainted. Wanting to see God touch his heart, I solicited the prayer support of my elderly mother on Bill's behalf. Sure enough, though fifteen years later, Bill became a Christian, became an active member of our church, and is one of the ministry shepherds who help me with the various ministries of the church.

Early one morning, while I was lying in my hospital bed, as clear as anything, God whispered to me, "Put a trailer hitch on your motorcycle. Have Bill do it." You need to understand that Pam and I enjoy motorcycle adventures. The fall before my leukemia experience, we had ridden the Appalachian Blue Ridge Parkway—390 miles with my sister and brother-in-law. It was wonderful, and I had lots of hopes and dreams for more adventures in the future. I had even made the statement that I wanted to "put a trailer hitch on my motorcycle so we could pull a trailer for long distance trips, like the Grand Canyon, or Yellowstone." I even dreamt of traveling the Alaska Highway to the forty-ninth state!

So, laying there in the pre-dawn darkness, with troubling questions buzzing through my brain, I heard God quietly whisper

101

to have Bill put a trailer hitch on my motorcycle. Like a sunrise, the message finally dawned. In another moment of my weakness, God was again assuring me that those traveling dreams were more than dreams. They were part of God's plan for me. Even though I didn't know how much time it was going to take for me to recover, or how God was going to heal me, those hopes, dreams, and plans were still intact. There was only one thing left to do—call Bill! So I called Bill and he and his wife reciprocated with a promised hitch and a hospital visit! Praise the Lord!

Assurance and encouragement are means the Comforter uses to deal with anxiety, doubt, and despair. But, like strapped on snowshoes, they can take you to newer, higher levels no matter how cold the chilly wind may blow. God was calling me and preparing me for a new spiritual level. And, in the next chapter, I'm going to address what God challenged me to do, two challenges that would sound foreign, or even crazy, to a lot of people.

Chapter 8

God's Challenge for Me . . .
Praise Him in the Storm and
Minister During the Storm

Though I was a very sick man, I was still a pastor. My first week in the hospital taught me in a fresh new way that sickness, no matter how serious, doesn't negate who we are. In fact, my sickness intensified my awareness that I was someone's husband, father, brother, and pastor. And this awareness, combined with my sickness, tempted me to allow the feelings of inadequacy, helplessness, and paralysis to overwhelm me. Satan, the evil one, doesn't refrain from temptation strategies because we are sick. Rather, he tends to pour it on, hoping that in our vulnerable moments, we will succumb. No wonder he is called the "evil one!"

In the prayer Jesus taught his disciples to pray, the proper translation of the phrase "and deliver us from evil," should be translated, "and deliver us from the evil one." Deliverance comes by trusting God and acting upon his promises. Therefore, the best counter strategy is simple faith in God's goodness and the willingness to act upon that faith. So, though I was a sick pastor, I was still a pastor. And my flock needed to hear from me. I took action.

During my first week in the hospital, I wrote a letter to my congregation and asked my prayer partner, Bryan Jaberg, to read it to them. In paraphrased form, it read as follows:

Dear Beloved Church Family:

I love you more than I ever have. God has stretched me more in the last week than I ever dreamed I could be stretched. This has been an incredible sorrow, but an incredible <u>blessing</u>, at the same time. Don't you <u>dare</u> let this make you question God or his faithfulness—"A righteous man's steps are ordered of the Lord"—even when they go through uncharted territory. Pam is a wonderful nurse. I've had some incredible visits from Jesus—He's the same God he has been on my 5-mile river walks. Something like this—a stunning shock like this—makes you reach way down inside and take ahold of all the truths you've preached . . . and guess what? . . . it is all true and it works! Everywhere I've been—every test I've had—every new room I've entered (fearfully) for treatments—I could see God went before me—I have so many stories to tell you in future sermons (if you don't mind listening to a skinny bald guy—ha).

If someone asks you how I am (yes, I'm deathly sick) but if someone asks you how I <u>really</u> am—tell them that I've never loved Jesus more—I never felt him closer—Jesus is the sweetest name I know. He <u>is</u> what <u>he says he is</u>. I love you with all of my heart.

Your pastor, friend,

Tom

P.S. Keep my office . . . I'm believing God for II Kings 20:1-6a

P.S.S. One of the greatest honors I had in my life was Thanksgiving Eve. Tommy, Scott, Allen & Kevin—Laid hands on me and all 4 prayed for my recovery.

Action! Faith *and* works! As I said in my letter, this was an incredible stretch for me. Though I had lived through a number of difficulties—the addiction of one son, the near death of another son, a nervous breakdown, and the trials and pressures of ministry—this experience was unique. This was a deeper time of despair than I had ever faced. God was calling my name, as I had preached in the *Day of Visitation* message. And, I felt that he was calling me to praise him during this time of storm. He was saying, "Tom, can you give me praise in the midst of this situation? Will you stretch further and minister for me during this situation?"

While pondering these questions, a popular gospel song began to play on my tape recorder. I will always thank God for this song by Casting Crowns:

> I'll praise You in this storm,
> And I will lift my hands.
> For You are who You are
> No matter where I am.
> Every tear I've cried
> You hold in Your hand;
> You never left my side.
> And though my heart is torn,
> I will praise You in this storm.

Covered with blood spots and in the midst of chemotherapy treatments, I was feeling as rough as I have ever felt. But, as Pam and I listened to this song, God, the Holy Spirit began to fill our room. Within seconds we felt his presence more intensely than we had ever experienced. As the vocalist sang "And I will lift my hands; for you are who you are, no matter where I am," God's presence was so powerful that I spontaneously raised my hands and began to praise him. Tears were running down my face as I began to praise the Lord amidst my sobbing. Instead of being swamped with the feelings of inadequacy, helplessness, and paralysis, I was overwhelmed with praise and thanksgiving for his faithfulness, realizing Romans 8:28 was really true—God works in all things for our good! Praising him in my storm was priming the pump for a continuing and sometimes cascading flow of blessing! Try, as I might, words fail me in describing what I felt in my heart and soul.

The moment passed, as the song concluded, but my hands remained raised, and my sobbing wouldn't cease. I glanced over to see my dear wife praising God in exactly the same way. All we can say is that something unique happened in our hospital room that day that neither one of us can explain. I don't know if God reached out his healing hand and touched me during this glorious praise experience. Perhaps he did, perhaps he didn't. What I do know is that I had a bone marrow test following that morning that showed unusual and exciting results. (I'll share that story a little later.) But, if I ever doubted before, I doubted no longer that "God works in mysterious ways, his wonders to perform!" And, I learned that the greatest joys come from praising God *during* the storms of life. I know this may sound irrational, even ludicrous to people who don't know Jesus Christ. But for the Christian believer, God's mysteries make perfect sense. Yes, we will praise Him for his faithfulness! Praise him for his goodness! Praise him for hardship! Praise him for difficulty! For the scriptures say, "Let everything that has breath, praise the Lord!"

Some may ask, "But I don't understand? Why does God want praise, especially when life is coming apart? Does he have a praise problem?" No, the problem is not his problem. Rather, the problem is our problem. God doesn't seek or need praise. He doesn't pace back and forth across the heavens wondering when we are going to praise him. Rather, when we praise God, we demonstrate that we are finally seeing life from an accurate, realistic, and proper perspective. When we praise God, we are acknowledging that he is God and we are not God. We are acknowledging that he is the creator and we are the creation, that he is infinite and we are finite, and that he is the Heavenly Father and we are his children. Praise is our acknowledgement of the great I AM. When we don't praise him, we ignore or disavow all of the above and our ability to see life clearly becomes limited and distorted. We become trapped in disappointments, delusion, and despair. We stumble about in a self-centered blindness, cursing our darkness.

But as our praise coupled with thanksgiving (gratitude), rises from our hearts, our hands, and our lips, his presence, like a glorious, dawn-illuminating sunrise, penetrates our darkness and bathes us with his light, his warmth, and his life Praise coupled with thanksgiving—a biblical couplet— opens our heart to God, just as it opens his heart to ours. Even in the midst of a life-threatening illness, I discovered that praising God opened my heart in a greater way to him, and he in turn, opened his heart in a greater way to me. The result: God took me to a new level of spiritual growth and maturity; he opened new doors for me; and he broke down some of the "strongholds" that had a grip on my life and ministry.

I want to elaborate on these statements a bit more. Like climbing a mountain, praising God in the midst of trial and storm will propel you to a new spiritual level. Mountain climbing isn't easy—especially with a heavy backpack—but it is worth it because you know the vistas are going to be spectacular! Or to use another metaphor, once you've been to 96th floor of the John Hancock building in Chicago, you are no longer content with what you can see on the 10th floor. You can see so much farther. You look from "above" instead of looking from "across." All the lower level glimpses are elevated to the magnificent beauty of the "big picture." In a similar way, God wants to take us to higher spiritual levels. And sometimes his means of doing this, or his "elevator," is praise—praise in the midst of a storm!

Last fall, as Pam and I motorcycled the Blue Ridge Parkway in the Appalachian Mountains, we would stop repeatedly at overlooks along the highway to drink in the breathtaking beauty of the vistas below. Stepping up to an overlook was like opening an unknown door on a whole new world. Photographs, paintings, or an IMAX movie are, at best, feeble attempts to capture what a "next level" personal view from an Appalachian overlook guarantees!

Praising God in the storm breaks strongholds. Strongholds are those experiences, events, and encounters that inhibit, intimidate, and restrict us from becoming all God wants us to be. Stronghold is another word for cage. Strongholds confine and shackle us. They can be things from our past—some ugliness from childhood, or experiences that ripped our heart in two. Scripture refers to "the pulling down" of strongholds. When we praise God in the midst of life's storms, we activate the "pulling down" process of God's liberating power. Jesus said, "You shall know the truth and the truth will set you free." Included in this truth is the understanding that our Heavenly Father is deserving of our praise regardless of our circumstances. He is to be honored and glorified. The practice of praise pulls down the strongholds of our past and sets us free!

I also learned that praising God in the storm is a way of teaching by example. I believe with all my heart that Christian believers are to teach by example. I should not call my congregation to do something I'm not willing to do myself. My personal spiritual growth must stay a step ahead if I'm to effectively help lead the way for others. Clear perspective has both a vertical *and* horizontal dimension. Thus, the Apostle Paul, in his letters of instruction to new believers says, "Be followers of me, as I am of Christ." Though Paul was human, far from perfect, and possessed flaws like the rest of us, he called his congregation to follow him, as he followed Christ.

As a result of the exceptional praise experience in my hospital room, and wanting to lead by example, I felt God prompting me to send another message to my congregation. Propped up on my hospital bed, I recorded the story of my praise experience via audio- tape, encouraging the congregation to open their hearts to the process of spiritual stretching, and challenged them to climb to a new spiritual level. The theme of my message was, "Praise God in the midst of the storm." Our assistant pastor agreed to play the tape during our Sunday worship service and then have Brandon Rouch, the young man who introduced me to the song *Praise You in this Storm,* sing it for the congregation. I asked that they stand while the song was being sung and praise the Lord for the storms in their lives.

The results were overwhelming. I was told by numerous people that the entire congregation stood to its feet, and with raised hands and tear-filled eyes, praised the Lord while Brandon sang this great song. Patti Thomas wrote me:

> *Oh what a mighty move of God's Spirit Sunday when we heard the song you requested, and everyone raised their hands in praise. Jim, my husband, raised both hands. The spirit was so sweet and definitely present. It was wonderful to hear that song. We are still continuing to pray for you.*

And Barbara, a dear woman who has recently walked through some very dark valleys—the suicide of her son (leaving a wife and two children), the death of her mother (cancer), and the death of her father—wrote that for the first time in her life, she praised God in a new way and at a new level. She said that during the singing of *Praise You in this Storm*, she stood, and with raised hands, praised God for her hardships. Such a demonstration would be out of character for Barb, a more reserved and quiet type person. I could tell from her letter, and from seeing her since then, that several "strongholds" had been pulled down. She was experiencing a new and liberating freedom. What an incredible witness to the church, for front-pew Barb to engage in such fervent praise to the Lord in the midst of her storms!

But, the sending of this second message to my congregation was just the beginning of God's plan for me to minister during my storm. Though I was learning to praise God in the midst of the storm, and learning to teach by example, I was still confined to a hospital room and virtually quarantined from society. I was sick, yes, very sick. And, I wondered, in my present and possibly future condition, could I still be who I am—a minister—in the midst of the greatest storm of my life?

I believe a minister is a servant. Sometimes reverends forget this. A servant just does one thing—serve. Oh, a person may have a title, travel the world, write a book, speak on the radio, and sermonize on TV, but if he doesn't serve, I don't think he is a minister. Serving others means offering them a cup of cold water in Jesus' name, preparing a meal, providing them with clothes, applying a healing balm to their wounds, lifting their spirit, and sharing the good news of the gospel of hope. I had always believed ministers were servants. My question was, "Did all this change because I was confined to a hospital?"

I was delighted when God spoke to my heart and said, "In addition to praising me in the storm, I want you to minister during this storm." And, the first opportunity to do so materialized very quickly.

At about 9:00 in the evening, Dr. Schultz was making his rounds and stopped by my room. I was feeling lousy and not prepared for much of a chat. The chemotherapy was taking its toll. My immune system was at a low level, my blood counts were dropping, and, though the staff didn't realize it at the time, I was having an allergic reaction to one of the antibiotic medications being pumped into me. My feet were on fire. They would itch to the place where I was almost frantic. I was more than weary of the endless regime of tests, chemotherapy, more tests, and innumerable medications.

Nevertheless, Dr Schultz stuck his head in the door and asked, "Would you do me a favor?" I had no idea of where he was going with this question. What kind of favor would he be asking of a very sick man at 9:00 o'clock at night?

Summoning an emotional second wind I said, "Sure."

He said, "I just admitted a young woman with leukemia. She's pregnant. I have to start chemotherapy immediately. I don't want to, but she won't live if I don't. Will you please pray for her?"

I said, "Absolutely."

Here it was! A marvelous opportunity to minister, to serve, in the midst of my storm! And, how affirming to have my doctor reveal his personal faith in the power of prayer! As he left the room, I got out of bed, rolled my IV stand over near the closet, grabbed a pillow for my knees (being vulnerable to severe bruising, I knelt with a pillow between my knees and the floor so I wouldn't bruise my knees), put my face on the bed, and began to pray for a woman I had never met. Pam joined me in prayer, kneeling at the adjacent couch. We had an extraordinary time of prayer, petitioning God to touch this young woman and be with her. God was present; both Pam and I sensed his presence in a powerful way. Any questions about being able to minister in the midst of storm evaporated. My hospital room had morphed into a sanctuary. It *was* possible to minister within the confining walls of a hospital room. Not only could one praise God in a storm, one could minister in a storm!

I later learned that the young lady's name was Mrs. Lee. Over a period of five months, she completed her treatment and fully recovered. She attributes her remission to prayer! Since then, I've had numerous chances to visit and pray with her in person. And, to reveal a little secret, I found that when we minister to others during our storms, it takes our eyes and mind off of ourselves. It reverses our tendencies to be selfish and self-centered, attitudes that can ferment into a brew of self-pity and despair.

During my subsequent rounds of chemotherapy, with my immune system strong enough so I could leave the room, I would push my IV pole from place to place visiting other patients. What a joy to see them respond to a cheery greeting or a word of encouragement! What a privilege to pray for people who were suffering with the same affliction I was suffering!

My room became a house of prayer. That in itself was a testimony to God's power. Sometimes, as people entered my room, they would remark that they sensed God's presence. Even the nurses were affected. I was amazed at how they responded to the Lord's presence and to me. A visiting doctor, filling in for Dr. Schultz, came by and said, "I've been wanting to meet you. I hear that you've been a blessing, and you're loved by all." While his words were complimentary, in his own way he was saying that he, and others, recognized that something unusual was happening in my room. God was present. He was helping me minister in the midst of my storm.

During my first hospital stay—a full 31 days in the same room—an idea was born that eventually came to full maturity. Because of the kindness of the St. Vincent doctors and 6th floor medical staff, I felt that I wanted to repay that kindness in some tangible way. I sensed that God was asking me to minister to cancer patients, as part of my pastoral ministry, for the rest of my life. When I expressed this thought to my doctor, he referred me to the woman in charge of the sixth floor, who referred me to the chaplain for the sixth floor. In our meeting, I asked if I could minister to cancer patients one day per week after I had fully recovered. To jump ahead in my story, that idea has come to full fruition. I currently spend one day (eight hours) each week on the sixth floor visiting with, and ministering to, cancer patients. Even so, I'll never be able to fully repay the goodness and graciousness that was shown to me.

Earlier in this chapter, I mentioned that during the incredible praise experience Pam and I shared in my hospital room, God may or may not have touched me with his healing hand. I don't know. I can't comprehend the greatness and goodness of an infinite God. What I do know is that the following morning's bone marrow test showed unusual and exciting results. But first, some context.

Immediately after I was admitted to the hospital on November 21, it seemed that nearly every day I would realize that the following phrase was echoing through my head: Twenty-one days; twenty-one days; twenty-one days. I was mystified and almost amused as I tried to figure out why this stream of consciousness kept repeating itself. I began to search the scriptures for references about anything related to twenty-one days, and discovered a most intriguing passage beginning in Daniel 10: 9. It reads like this:

I heard Him speaking, and then I listened. A hand touched me and set me trembling on my hands and knees. He said, "Daniel, you are highly esteemed. Consider carefully the words I am about to speak to you. Now stand up for I have now been sent to you."

When He said this to me, I stood up, trembling. Then He continued, "Do not be afraid, Daniel. Since the first day that you set your mind to understand and to humble yourself before God your words were heard. And I have come to respond to them. But the Prince of Persia Kingdom resisted me 21 days. Then Michael the Archangel came and helped me."

As I read that passage, I had an exceedingly strong sense that there was something significant in this scriptural passage for me. I read it again. It seems Daniel was praying earnestly about issues regarding his future, among other things. Nothing happened until God sent an angel to Daniel who acknowledged Daniel prayer, but stated that the answer was held up for twenty-one days due to resistance from the Prince of Persia (an evil power). But on the twenty-second day, Michael, the Archangel (an even greater power) was sent by God to answer Daniel's prayer.

Because the phrase twenty-one days had repeatedly come to mind, and the passage in Daniel resonated with something in my spirit, I told my wife that I had the feeling something significant was going to happen on the twenty-second day of my hospital stay. That belief was based upon my comments at the very beginning of this chapter about the strategy and power of the evil one. I believed that, as a servant/minister, I was experiencing more than a physical sickness. I felt that the evil one had a hand in this storm I was experiencing and was challenging our ministry, and, perhaps, even attempting to destroy it. I later discovered that several others felt the same way, and were fervently praying and fasting on my behalf. This was about something more than a rural pastor from central Indiana developing leukemia!

Twenty-one days. What did that mean? I waited as the days went by; continuing to wonder what would happen on the twenty-second day. Twenty-one days would be December 11. I wondered what December 12 would hold?

On the morning of December 12, Dr. Schultz came into my room with the world's biggest smile on his face. In an excited, joyful voice he said, "You should be a poster boy for Acute Myeloid Leukemia recovery! The resilience you are having with this chemotherapy is incredible! I highly suspect you are already in full remission. What's more, you are going to be discharged in the next few days and can receive your next round of chemo as an outpatient. Those rounds will only be precautionary, for it appears that the cancer cells are gone!"

What a glorious twenty-second day! I wept with joy! All praise to God the Father, God the Son, and God the Holy Spirit!

After thanking the Lord, I expressed my gratitude for Dr. Schultz and his marvelous team, continuing to be impressed that every time he gave me any news, he acknowledged that God was in control. I remember as I thanked him again and again, he would point up and say, "We had help."

I have no idea why, early on, God whispered twenty-one days in my ear. I just know he did. Equally amazing, and without knowing any of the above, Chris Edgington, our children's pastor, who filled the pulpit each week during this same twenty-one day period I was in the hospital, preached a sermon about how an evil force resisted and delayed the answer to Daniel's prayer, and how, at the end of twenty-one days, Daniel prayer was answered. All I can conclude is that our faithful, loving, Heavenly Father was alerting us to the strategy of the evil one. Our God is amazing! The leading of his Holy Spirit is astonishing!

Chapter 9

Going Bald

It might seem a little strange, after sharing spiritual truths and encouraging letters of comfort from friends, to title a chapter, "Going Bald." While I'm going to tell you the full story of how losing my hair impacted me, I chose this title for another reason.

For me, and I think for others like me, the process of losing one's hair brings the reality of cancer home to roost like nothing else. Many of us may remember our first reaction upon seeing a beloved relative in a hospital room as a hairless cancer patient. It is hard to fully control one's surprise or alarm at the sight of no eyebrows, a shiny scalp, and, in some cases, no body hair of any kind. As we looked at them, and tried to absorb their difference in appearance, we recognized the reality of cancer and the devastation of its treatment. While improved medications help lessen nausea, high temperatures, etc., there are some side effects that cannot be helped. Chemotherapy is poison, and as I understand it, chemotherapy kills the cancerous cells *and* everything else in the blood. What medical experts do, is give the patient a drug strong enough to kill everything, then replace the killed cells with live cells through endless transfusions of new blood and blood platelets. My temperature hovered in the 102° F range, spiking to 105 due to an infection. With an immune system close to zero, my situation was a very dangerous one.

But, it is also important to address the emotional trauma of chemotherapy. The poison filtering through one's body is also filtering through one's brain. It affects your thinking, and your emotions. As I received high doses of Ara-C and Idarubisin, I probably experienced more traumas emotionally than I did physically. This type of trauma is not explained very well in the pre-treatment booklets you are given to read. Because each of us is unique chemically, it may be hard to generalize on what should or shouldn't happen when it comes to emotion.

I was overwhelmed with insecurity. This frightened me since I've always been a fairly confident person. I've always been pretty sure of my gifts and abilities. For example, during the two weeks I was out of the hospital over Christmas, I was baffled at how fearful I was to play the guitar in front of the congregation. I've played the guitar in front of people for 35 or 40 years. I'm usually very comfortable standing in front of people. But now, I would have short panic attacks while starting a song, wondering if I could remember the guitar chords. I was afraid, experiencing a fear brought on by the trauma of chemotherapy treatments.

Fear affects all areas of life. I would have fear if Pam left the room. She was very faithful to stay by my side, but if she left the room and was gone for a few minutes, I would become very uneasy. While I knew this fear created tremendous pressure for her, it didn't lessen the fear. Three weeks into my treatment, Pam felt she needed to go back to our home in Logansport and wash some clothes and pay our monthly bills. Knowing this was a sensible thing for her to do, I still struggled with fear even though I knew she would be back that evening. My emotional trauma was only exacerbated when the TV news said to expect heavy snowfall from a sizeable Midwest storm.

But, it was a good struggle. God uses different means to stretch us. Scripture became incredibly important to me, for much of the Bible, especially the book of Psalms, addresses fear. "Fear not, for I am with you" is said in many places and in many ways. And, as I searched the scriptures, God helped me face my fears. He affirmed that he is "a very present help in time of trouble." He is our refuge. His everlasting arms are beneath us. We might think we're falling, but his arms are there to catch us!

I remember getting a card from a woman at church named Joyce. It's no coincidence that it came on the morning Pam left for home. The card said:

The one who has been with you this far will not let you down now.

Keep trusting!

It was a message from the Lord! He was saying, "Tom, you are safe. The hospital is prepared for storms, the nurses are nearby, Pam possesses good judgment, and your friends are telling you to 'keep trusting.' Tom, relax!" That afternoon, prompted by the Holy Spirit, Dr. Fraiz, a devoted Christian, stopped by for a chat. He sat down on my bed, and in a very relaxed manner, visited with me for 30 minutes. I immediately realized how unusual this visit from a very busy doctor really was. It, too, was a gift from God.

While God helped me with my fears, I noticed that I was experiencing other emotional side effects from the chemotherapy. My reservoirs for emotional stability and control were very low. I have always been one who could multi-task. That changed after the chemotherapy treatments started. If I was talking to someone, and the phone would ring (two things occurring at the same time), I would almost go to pieces emotionally. The level at which I became overwhelmed by the normal occurrences of life was much lower than I had ever experienced. And, these changes, both emotionally and physically, happened so fast. I think it would be helpful if doctors could explain this better to patients so they could anticipate this kind of emotional upheaval.

While all the prescribed treatments can produce uncertainty and anxiety, looking into a mirror to see baldness is a reality check! Like my father (who had all of his hair until he died at 89 years of age), I have always been blessed with a thick head of hair. Baldness doesn't exist among the Robbins men. Back in the 70's, I even wore my hair longer, down over my ears, and combed back. People complimented me on my hair. I also had a full beard that I kept neatly trimmed. I was a man with a lot of hair on my face and head.

It was a moment to remember, when my hair began to fall out. It quickly became patchy. I would wake up and there would be hair on my pillow. I would comb through my hair, and there would be wads of hair in my comb. I would wash my hair and there would be balls of hair in the sink. I tried to joke with people by telling them I was beginning to look like a possum— blotchy and mangy. But, every time I looked into a mirror I realized what this devastating disease and its treatment was doing to me, and how it was affecting me and changing me. I actually considered shaving my head, but thought I'd wait a few more days. I guess I was trying to hang on to what looked like me for a little while longer.

Once again, the Lord arranged to give my spirit a major boost. My sister Miriam has always been close to me. Paul, Jim, Sharon, and Caroll (who died as an adult) were all older siblings. (Paul was a college freshman when I was born.) Miriam was just 30 months older; we grew up together. I don't think one could have a better sister. During this time of emotional and physical trauma, Miriam came to see me. As she walked into my room I noticed that she was bundled up in a heavy winter coat and a big, floppy hat. Since it was December, I didn't think much about her apparel, although it was unusual for Miriam to wear a hat. She came over to my bed, leaned down, and kissed me on the cheek and said, "Tom, I love you, and I want to identify with you."

As I looked up, wondering what she meant, she majestically jerked her hat off, revealing a completely shaved head! Wow! My sister, a very attractive woman, with a shaved head! I'm not usually at a loss for words, but I was stunned into total silence. When I could finally put some words together, I stammered,

"Well, I knew you loved me, but I didn't realize you loved me this much!"

Miriam has always had gorgeous, jet-black hair. She obviously has some of the Robbins' family hair genes. She styles her hair beautifully, as part of her always well-groomed appearance. Since she is one of the worship leaders at her church (and up in front of hundreds of people) she makes it a point to look as nice as possible. Now, here in my room, on a cold, winter day, with all of the Christmas season activities of her church looming before her, she stood before me completely bald, saying she cared enough about me to identify with me! Knowing that I had always had great hair, and that it would be hard for me to lose my hair, she looked for a way to make my loss easier for me.

If I had to list one-time, simple acts of kindness that have had a great effect on me, I would put Miriam's shaved head on that list. It was an incredible thing for her to do. In fact, the following Christmas Sunday, when I had the privilege of speaking to my congregation, I told them the story of Miriam shaving her head, and how her desire to identify with me reminded me of the love of Jesus. I pointed out that the reason Jesus left the glories of heaven, and came to earth as a babe in a manger, was to identify with us. Miriam not only identified with me, she gave me great sermon material!

A couple of days following Miriam's visit, I shaved my head. My hair got to the point where I was looking quite hideous. So I propped myself up in front of the bathroom mirror and sink and went to work. My wife, waiting to see what I looked like, called through the door, "How does it look?"

I said, "I look like Kojak with E. T.'s ears." I've always been self-conscious about my large ears. She got a kick out of my quip.

If you ever want someone to pray for you, my wife should be the one to ask. I often tease her with that statement because of her prayers for me. She didn't tell me until two months later, but she prayed that I wouldn't lose my mustache. She knew that, having had a full head of hair and a full beard and mustache, losing everything would be quite an adjustment for me. And, after three rounds of intense chemotherapy, I never completely lost my mustache. No one could believe it. I lost all of my scalp hair, and my entire beard, but I retained a small mustache.

During this time of loss, I received a very special letter from a friend named Mark that gave me a great laugh. Here is a paraphrased version:

Tom,

In the letter your prayer partner read to the church, you made the statement, "I hope you don't mind listening to a skinny bald guy preach." I have been thinking about how God has used baldness to initiate growth in people. Even in secular situations, people have benefited from the loss of hair.

The Bible says God blessed Samson from the time of his youth. But did he ever really seek God or have the humility that he should, until he had no hair and little strength? He grew to depend on God because he had nothing else, and received God's strength after hitting bottom.

I can't remember any of Ernest Borgnine's films when he had hair. Fame came when his hair was gone. Kojak! Now there's a perfect example of a man with hair that couldn't find a major acting part! So, he shaved his head for a reading, got the part, and became the TV actor of his time!

Let's look at sports. Who is the greatest basketball player of this generation and, arguably, ever? A bald guy in Chicago! Michael Jordan had hair in high school and was cut from his team. He had hair at North

122

Carolina and played in the shadow of James Worthy and Sam Perkins. He had hair when he was drafted fourth behind number one Sam Bowie. (Sam must have never shaved his head because he disappeared from the scene even though he had a lot of potential.) Jordan struggled the first couple of years, and then shaved his head. The rest is a history of NBA titles. I wonder how much better Larry Bird could have been if he had been bald?

Top ten scorers of NBA history: Kareem Abdul Jabar--bald, Carl Malone--bald, Oscar Robertson, still has hair; too bad, he could have been number one, Michael Jordan--bald, Wilt Chamberlain (I think he ended up bald), Charles Barkley--bald, Julius Irving--afro to bald--got better as he went along, George Garvin--bald, and Reggie Miller--bald!

I, myself, never felt close to God until five years ago when I shaved my head for my own security reasons. Huh? I'm seeing a pattern here?

I doubt that Tom Robbins would ever have shaved his head, but God is going to use Tom's baldness as another opportunity for him to be all that he can be. Huh? "Be all that you can be!" Isn't that a slogan of the US Army? Recruits have their heads shaved at the very beginning of basic training! Every famous evangelist I can think of has hair. Move over Billy Graham (who still has lots of hair), Tom Robbins may well be on his way to the number one spot. Just something for you to think about, my dear friend.

We love and miss you!

Mark

How clever! How thoughtful that Mark would have the sensitivity to send me a letter saying he is praying and caring for me while providing me with a good laugh!

However, as is so often true during chemotherapy treatment, I went from a moment of laughter to what felt like a D-Day experience. I can't adequately express in words the anxiety that gripped me when Dr. Schultz came to my room to do a bone marrow test. What was going on in my bone marrow would tell the medical experts a lot about where I was physically, and what needed to be done in the future. It was my D-Day. Few were optimistic, even though they were mystified by how well I was responding to treatment.

Performed in my room, the test consisted of injecting a very large needle into my hipbone to extract bone marrow. To accomplish this, a great deal of pressure must be placed upon the needle. The test is intimidating and painful. Then it takes three days to analyze the marrow to see what is going on and to determine the future course of treatment. The waiting time is filled with uncertainty.

Most people, who have leukemia at the advanced stage of my disease, would need a bone marrow transplant, if a transplant would work at all. But, in spite of the uncertainty and the pessimism of others, I was feeling optimistic. I was claiming the verses that God had given me. I was doing well, compared to how most people do in this situation. I remember looking across at my wall and reading the verses from II Kings as the bone marrow test was being performed:

I will heal you, and I will add 15 years to your life.

What a comfort that was! Yet, I must admit that, physically, I still was experiencing quite a bit of anxiety.

Two and a half days later I received a phone call on a Saturday. I will always be indebted to Dr. Schultz for seeing to it that the call was made. He could have easily waited until Monday, but he had a team member call on a Saturday afternoon. In an excited voice, the doctor who called said, "I've got some great news. The bone marrow test came back very, very good." I didn't know until Monday, when Dr. Schultz explained it to me, exactly what the test revealed. His exact words on Monday were, "There are no residual cancer cells showing in the bone marrow." It was amazing! These results were occurring only three weeks after treatment had begun, three weeks after my white count had been 137,000 and I was covered with blood spots and bleeding from between my teeth and from my nose! Everyone was surprised by these results.

What an amazing blessing! I don't know, even now, that I grasp the full extent of this "great news." I still sometimes struggle with feelings of guilt and unworthiness, knowing that so many people receive "bad news" after their medical tests have been administered. I don't understand, nor can I explain why God gave me His word and wanted, for some reason, to add years to my life. All I know for sure is that I had come to a place of accepting his will, whether it was life or death. My life belonged to the Lord to do as he saw fit.

Dr. Schultz determined that, despite the good bone marrow test, I needed to go ahead with treatment. Though I mentioned to him that I was a little concerned as to why we were going to do more treatment after hearing that my bone marrow was cancer free, knowing more treatment would take a tremendous toll on me, I submitted to his judgment. You may recall that when I first had prayer with Dr. Schultz, I said I was going to submit to what my doctor told me to do. Dr. Schultz decided it would be foolish not to continue treatment as a preventative measure. I submitted to his decision fully and completely.

I believe God puts people in special places of authority. I believe God is at work when we don't understand why, what, when, and how. Even though God had given me his word about healing, my doctor felt that I should continue treatment. I knew submission was the right choice. However, Dr. Schultz said he was going to try to get me out of the hospital for the week of Christmas, before I began a second set of treatments. With my immune system near zero, we would wait for it to rebuild, and then I would have a final high-dose treatment requiring hospitalization.

So, here it was: December! Chemotherapy was taking its toll. My immune system was near zero and I had to be extremely cautious about contact with other people. In fact, I was quarantined to my room. Everyone needed to wear a mask and wash their hands repeatedly before they came into my room.

But, I had the Lord, and I had hope. I hoped that my immune system would rebuild fast enough for me to have the privilege of attending a Christmas service at my church. That was my goal. And, Christmas fell on Sunday. Wasn't it neat that Christmas day was on a Sunday? (It happens once every seven years or so.) I was looking forward to seeing my congregation.

Chapter 10

Home for Christmas—What a Blessing!

Many of us struggle with the question of whether God answers prayer. We shouldn't, but we do. I believe that God always answers prayer—in his own time, and in his own way. And when he answers, he usually does far more for us than we have asked, or even knew to ask! In Scripture we read, "Now unto him who is able to do exceedingly, abundantly above all that we ask or think (Ephesians 4:20a)." The problem we often bring to prayer is the problem of our own agenda, the way in which we feel prayer should be answered. When our prayers aren't answered in the way we expected, we assume God didn't answer. The truth is, God answers prayer, and usually does it a way that exceeds anything we could possibly ask.

As a young man I asked God to help me be a good pastor. I prayed that he would help me be a good leader and a good example. My desire was to help people grow and develop. That is what pastoring is supposed to be. Little did I realize that God would use leukemia as a means of answering my prayer. From a strictly human perspective, I could have viewed my sickness as a "time out," a time away from the church, and a time when others would fill the gap. Certainly, our pastoral staff did a wonderful job in my absence. But, what I discovered is that I had more impact on the congregation through my illness than I did when I was present and well. It is so amazing how God answers prayer in ways we didn't expect!

During my weeks in the hospital, there were hundreds of confirmations that God was answering my prayer. Some were right to the point. People like Irma Moshesh, who has battled cancer herself, told me that she sensed, while praying for me, that my hospitalization was about more than just leukemia. Rather, it was for the development of my congregation.

I received a card from Josh's family. I don't know Josh's last name, but three years ago, while visiting Milwaukee, Wisconsin, on one of our motorcycle trips, I felt prompted by the Holy Spirit to visit a family who was having a yard sale to raise funds to help pay for their son's cancer treatment. Josh was very much disabled with cancer. We visited the sale. Though we were total strangers, I sensed we should stop and pray for Josh. For some reason, I had taken a small bottle of anointing oil with me. As I look back, it was seems odd to me that I would take anointing oil along, but I did. After introducing ourselves and establishing some social rapport, we made a circle and anointed and prayed for Josh.

Later, they sent me a family picture saying God had touched Josh, and he was doing very well. Now, they sent a card saying they were praying for me! This small gesture of kindness was an incredible encouragement to me while I was hoping to go home for Christmas.

The confirmation that touched me the most deeply came from my father. However, this anecdote requires a bit of context. I mentioned earlier that my father was an amazingly godly man. He had a prophet's anointing. An excellent speaker, he seemed to stand head and shoulders above others in his understanding and articulation of the scriptures.

At the time of my hospitalization, Dad was in a healthcare center in Warren, Indiana, struggling with dementia. After Mother died, we had tried to keep him in his own home, but escalating medical problems and failing mental function required the 24-hour specialized care only professionals can provide. Even before he died, we grieved that he no longer knew us or remembered us. Communication with him seemed no longer possible. We couldn't have been more wrong!

Shortly after Mother died, and while he still had some mental capacity, Dad sent a handwritten portion of Psalm 40 to Patty Gibbs, an active member of our congregation. When she opened the letter, she just found some scripture verses—no personal note, no explanation, just some verses from Psalm 40. Though Patty was aware of Dad's failing mind, she was still mystified by his letter. She read the verses several times, wondering what they meant and how they might apply to her, wondering why he had sent them to her. Because Patty had developed a lot of confidence in Dad through the years, she sensed that this scripture had great significance of some kind, but she couldn't figure out what it was. As the weeks went by she filed the letter away and forgot about it.

Five years later, when she heard that I was in the hospital with leukemia, she remembered Dad's letter, and immediately wondered if the letter had something to do with me. She retrieved it and read it again. This time it all made perfect sense to her. God was speaking through the Psalmist (and my father) with a much-needed affirmation for me. Even with a failing mind, Dad still had his prophet's anointing, and he knew that sometime in the future I would need these verses from Psalm 40:1-3:

> *I waited patiently for the Lord; and He inclined to me, and heard my cry. He brought me up out of a slimy pit, out of the mud and mire, and set my feet on a rock. He gave me a firm place to stand. He put a new song in my mouth—a hymn of praise to our God. Many will see, and fear, and put their trust in the Lord.*

What a remarkable message from my prophetic father! Unable to verbally communicate with me, he somehow managed to send an affirmation/confirmation to Patty five years before I would need it. How faithful God is! And what was the affirmation/confirmation? Verse three: "Many will fear (show reverence for God)," it says, "and put their trust in the Lord." As I've mentioned, this verse was fulfilled hundreds of times, as I witnessed how God touched lives during my illness. The letters and cards just kept coming, as people let me know how God was dealing with them because of my illness.

The hardest part of my hospitalization was the waiting. Waiting is hard work! What helped were my hopes that I would be home in time for Christmas. My immune system became stronger with each passing day. It finally reached a point of enough strength that Dr. Schultz dropped by and announced, "You're going to get to go home for Christmas—actually, five days before Christmas." This news brought a combination of great joy and deep sadness to my heart. While I felt exceedingly privileged to be able to go home, I knew there were other cancer patients on the sixth floor who would not be going home for Christmas.

The day of departure arrived, a cold, winter's day, but nevertheless a blessed day! Pam parked our car near the hospital entrance, and with the help of one of the nurses, she carried my personal things to the car. I stayed in the room, and for the first time in 31 days, I put on some street clothes. It felt strange to sit there alone in the room. I paused, and bowed my head and thanked the Lord for all the experiences and blessings he had given me in that room. Even though I was thrilled with the idea of going home, when I stepped out of the room and looked down the long hospital corridor, I was gripped with a panic-like fear. The emotional trauma that often accompanies chemotherapy raced through me like an adrenalin rush! I felt incredibly insecure about leaving what had been my safe place for the last 31 days. The insecurity was so real that I gripped Pam and said, "I'm afraid. I'm afraid to leave the room." Reason and emotion collided head on, as they sometimes do. I knew I shouldn't be afraid; I didn't expect to be afraid; but I was afraid!

We walked down the hall and got on the elevator complete with a bald head draped in a facemask. I tried to keep from standing too close to other people in the elevator, for my immune system levels were 0.5. Though it was a low number, my doctor felt if was good enough to let me go home as long as I was careful about personal contact. Before we left the building, I told Pam that I wanted to stop at the hospital chapel for a prayer of thanksgiving. Praying in the chapel was a moment I'll never forget. I had stopped there many times before to pray for the needs of other people, as a part of my pastoral care responsibilities. Now, I was thanking God for his goodness to me, and for the privilege of going home.

We got in the car and headed home. It was so strange to go north on US Highway 31 and look at very familiar scenes, as though I were seeing them for the very first time. I continued to struggle with feelings of insecurity. I began to understand why people who are quarantined, or are confined in concentration camps don't always leave when offered the opportunity. How quickly we adjust to the "security" of a smaller, more familiar world and try to avoid the larger, more unfamiliar world!

After a two-hour ride, we started up the road where I had walked and prayed for several years. I was flooded with so many wonderful memories of talking with the Lord during my prayer walks. But, I was also aware that my life had changed in major ways since I had last prayer-walked this road. I would never be the same. I was riding down this road a changed person.

My wife had called ahead to tell Scott that we were coming. He had asked to be notified since he wanted to do something special for me as a "welcome home" gift. Scott knew that among our horses, Cody, who is very responsive to me, was my favorite. So, as we drove up the driveway, there stood our four quarter horses, including Cody. I admit that I wondered if Cody would recognize a no-hair me, even though I had a sock hat pulled down over my ears. As we pulled up next to the barn, Scott was sitting on the fence smiling. He had put some hay on the ground to keep the horses milling around in the driveway as we parked and got out of the car. I immediately walked up to Cody and called him by name. He looked at me for a moment, jerked his head slightly in a horse-like acknowledgement, and then nickered a greeting! That may seem like a small thing to you, but for me, it was the beginning of a connection with a world larger than a hospital room.

Among all of the lessons I learned from my leukemia experience, the lesson of connecting with the "little things" in life became one of the more valuable ones. We need to appreciate every moment of every day. Little connections, little acts of kindness, little greetings, even if it is the nicker of a horse, have great value! God, who is aware of every sparrow that falls, puts a high premium on little things.

I was overwhelmed with emotion, though in a detached sort of way, as I walked into the house. I stood and stared at the living room, where I always sat and studied, and at the kitchen where I had spent many delightful moments. It seemed that I had entered another world. Feeling like a stranger in my own home, I kept looking for more ways to connect. It continued to confuse me that I was still emotionally tethered to my hospital room. I wanted to be home, I knew this was my home and I needed to be here, but a full connection to home was still beyond my grasp.

Scott suggested that I go to the telephone answering machine and press the play button. As I responded to his suggestion, I heard the soft, raspy voice of Matt Hunt, a wheelchair confined quadriplegic who finds it difficult to speak because of a permanent tracheotomy tube say, "Welcome home Tom. I know what it's like to be in the hospital and then get to come home." Between my favorite horse's nicker and a prayer partner's raspy voice I was beginning to sense that God knew all about my adjustment struggle, and he would help me find the tangible connections I needed for the next chapter of life.

My first evening went well. Because Pam had come home the day before to decorate the house and trim a tree, I spent the evening sitting by the lighted tree feeling the "Spirit of Christmas" settling down over me. Over and over I told Pam how absolutely wonderful it was to sit by a Christmas tree in my own home. The next day Dr. Schultz called to wish me a Merry Christmas. As I recall, he said, "Tom, I'm calling to wish you and your family a Merry Christmas. I trust things are going well for you, and I'm sure your congregation will be glad to see you on Sunday." Dr. Schultz had worked especially hard to build my immune system to the place that I could be in church on Christmas Sunday with my congregation. He knew it would mean a lot to me to be with them on this very special day. He also thanked me for a plaque I had given him that spoke of my gratitude for him as a doctor, and for the way God had used him to spare my life. A friend had made that plaque for me while I was in the hospital.

The next morning I sensed I was doing better, but I still didn't feel quite at home. This bothered me greatly, because I've always loved my home, knowing it was a gift from the Lord (a story in itself). So I asked the Lord, "What should I do? I need to reconnect." God heard my prayer and spoke to me in my spirit. It wasn't an audible voice, but I had a very clear impression that I should reconnect with the last things I did before I left home to go to the hospital. I told Pam that I was going to bundle up, wear a sock hat and a mask, and go outside for a walk. I felt I should retrace my last deer hunting steps in early November, the week before my leukemia diagnosis. I would advise anyone who is feeling estranged or disconnected, as I was, to reconnect with things familiar to you. Force yourself to do things and revisit places that will connect you with your former world. That world can continue to seem like a dream world once you leave the hospital, if you don't reconnect as soon as possible.

I remember walking slowly through the pasture and the wooded area adjacent to it, past the tree where I had stood in the deer stand. I let myself remember how God had spoken to me about the deer. I walked to the fence and looked out over the area where I had collapsed and fallen to the snow-covered ground. From there I walked back to the lot next to our house where the horses always stand in the winter. I walked up to Cody, took hold of his halter, and began petting him on the face. He quickly nuzzled up next to me as I continued to pet his face. I began to sob and cry. All the desire for wellness, wholeness, and longing for home flooded through me in an expression of sobs and tears. I truly and finally reconnected with the world of home, sweet home. I probably cried harder than I've cried for years, and Cody, who seemed to understand in some way what I was feeling, just stood there nuzzled up next to me. It may sound ridiculous, but I believe this simple scenario of a bald-headed man in a sock hat, hanging on to a horse, crying his eyes out, was God ordered and directed. It was God's way of preparing me for what was to come.

As an aside, I would like to say that one of the miracles and blessings God puts on earth for us is animals. I think we often overlook the obvious. God has often used animals in my life to speak to me, to direct me, to comfort me. Petting my horse and revisiting the place where I had encountered the deer provided a connection with God and real life that all the graciousness of so many wonderful people didn't fully provide. I don't fully understand everything I'm saying here, but I know I felt very much at home for the first time since my hospitalization after this intense, personal experience.

The next day, feeling I needed to think through my upcoming Christmas sermon, I decided to take another walk. As I was ambling along, I heard a truck coming up behind me. As I turned around, I could see that it was my neighbors, Glen and Donna Hall. Donna has battled cancer for a number of years and must be treated periodically through the port in her chest. Seeing them touched my heart, because I knew Donna would identify with what I was experiencing. I wasn't sure they would recognize me since I looked quite different then when I had last walked this road. But, they obviously did, and as they pulled up beside me, I could see that Glen had tears in his eyes. He greeted me, and then said, "I just told Donna, 'Now, that's a familiar sight—Tom walking and praying.'" Glen had driven by and waved to me dozens of time in the past. I had no idea he was aware that I was praying as I walked. I was touched by his comment and realized once again that one's neighbors do notice how you live. I feel great love for Glen and Donna. We are blessed to have such good neighbors.

I continued to prepare for Christmas Sunday. Having learned something about reconnecting at home, I felt the acute necessity to reconnect with my church as well. Friday evening I asked my son Kevin, to take me over to the church so I could rehearse the song *Give Me Jesus*. It was the song I wanted to sing my first day back in the pulpit. While I've always been a singer, and had sung this song many times before, I wondered if the chemotherapy treatment had affected my voice to the place where trying to sing a song with an accompaniment tape, recorded in a fairly high key, was out of the question. I also felt the need to physically reconnect with the church environment, with the sanctuary and the platform setting, rather than being overwhelmed by the "newness" of everything Christmas Sunday morning. I didn't want to feel detached from the physical environment as I stood in front of my congregation for the first time.

It was wonderful to walk into an empty church, step up to the platform, and stand in front of the microphone with my guitar strapped around my shoulder. After rehearsing for some time, I knew I would be able to sing the song. I'll always appreciate the hour and a half I had with Kevin that evening, as I rehearsed *Give Me Jesus,* and he played sound engineer.

Christmas Sunday morning arrived! Pam and Kevin left early to rehearse with the praise band. Since my immune system resistance was still lower than normal, Kevin agreed to "stand in my place" as the praise band rehearsed so I could arrive just before the worship service began. Tom, our firstborn, had agreed to drive me to the church. On our way there, I didn't say anything to Tom, but I will admit I was nervous. I knew Christmas morning is a very special time for many families, a time to gather together and celebrate this wonderful holiday by the giving of gifts. I wondered if attendance would be down, and whether people would delay or postpone their family traditions in order to participate in our worship service. I had reason to believe some of my closest friends would be there, for they had heard that I was home from the hospital.

As we approached the church (I still feel the emotion of this moment), I realized that the parking lot was full, with additional cars parked out on the road. Every available seat in the church was taken. It was filled to capacity. There were folding chairs up and down the aisles. Even the hallways were packed. It was standing room only! I don't ever remember seeing our church that full. I was blown away as I slipped in a side door adjacent to the platform. It was important that I not encounter people directly because of my weakened immune system. Handshakes and hugs were out of the question.

As planned, I walked out onto the platform after Chris Edgington, our children's pastor led the children's choir in an opening Christmas carol. When the people saw me, after my "surprise" entrance, the entire congregation stood in praise to God and began to applaud. I was so humbled by their response that I went to my knees in tears as they continued to applaud and praise the Lord!

The moment called for more than tears, so I did the first thing that came to my mind. I stood to my feet, grinned at the congregation, grabbed the sock hat I was wearing, and jerked it off. There was an audible gasp, peals of laughter, and thunderous applause. I will never forget the expressions on the faces of the first three rows of teenagers when they saw me completely hairless. After the moment had run its course, I stepped up to the pulpit and spent the next several minutes thanking everyone for such tremendous love and support. I told them that no pastor had ever had a congregation that loved him as much as they did. Then I began to sing, *Give Me Jesus*.

Though I had sung this song many times before, *Give Me Jesus* took on a whole new meaning for me this special Christmas morning:

> ***In the morning, when I rise, give me Jesus.***
>
> ***When I am alone, give me Jesus.***
>
> ***When I come to die, give me Jesus.***
>
> ***You can have all this world, but give me Jesus.***

137

Then Pam, Marilyn Rouch, and I sang the chorus *In Jesus' Name We Press On*. I remember exchanging glances with Pam as we sang, both of us realizing what we had just been through together:

> *In Jesus' name, we press on,*
>
> *In Jesus' name, we press on;*
>
> *Dear Lord, with the prize clear before our eyes,*
>
> *We find the strength to press on.*

We finished with the refrain of the wonderful gospel song, *Jesus Is the Sweetest Name I Know*. Every one of these songs came from my heart, for Jesus *had* become the sweetest name I had ever known.

Kevin stepped forward, and with the backing of the praise band, fervently led the congregation in singing:

> *You are mighty,*
>
> *You are holy,*
>
> *You are awesome in your power.*
>
> *You have risen,*
>
> *You have conquered,*
>
> *You have beaten the power of death.*

Until I heard the congregation respond like a mighty choir, it didn't dawn on me how powerful the message of this song is for a Christmas Sunday morning. It was a glorious morning of praise, honor, and worship to the "babe in the manger, who is the King of Glory." Only a worship service in heaven would be more glorious!

We completed the service and I slipped out the side door to head home for a family Christmas dinner. How blessed could a man be, especially one recovering from a potentially fatal illness?

I still couldn't believe I was home with my family, as well as with my church, for Christmas Sunday! We sat at the dinner table—Pam, each of our four sons, and our wonderful daughter-in-law, Trisha—thanking the Lord for his goodness to us! A highlight was being able to hold my grandson, Braxten. The doctors had said that it would be permissible to have contact with my family within the confines of our home, since my immune system was conditioned to them. It was in public places where I needed to be most careful.

Braxten was 18 months old, and we enjoyed many grandpa/grandson activities appropriate for his age including "pretend" motorcycle riding. He would stand on my lap facing me, while I would put out my two index fingers like they were motorbike handlebars. Braxten would wrap his little fingers around my index fingers, and pretend he was riding a motorcycle, complete with sound effects. At first he was a little hesitant to play when he saw me without a sock hat. He would ask, "Pawpaw?" He knew he was hearing Pawpaw's voice, but my voice didn't match his memory of my appearance. However, it wasn't long before we reconnected through pretend motorcycle, "horsey" rides on my back, and a host of other activities.

The days between Christmas and New Years' sped by quickly. I had been advised to watch very closely for fevers and other signs of respiratory infections. A common cold can turn into a medical emergency when one's immune system has been compromised by chemotherapy. I had also been advised that a second set of chemotherapy treatments would be required for preventive reasons as soon as my immune system could handle the stress. After the second set of treatments, I would take another break while my immune system recovered, and then finish with a "high-dose" treatment sometime in March.

Even though I was a "treatment veteran," I felt a wave of anxiety as I contemplated the rigors of another round of chemotherapy. As I've heard others say, "Chemotherapy sure beats death, but not by much!" I sensed that the evil one was harassing me with fear about the forthcoming "treatment time" despite all the wonderful things that had happened to date. I asked God to give me another assurance that everything was under his control. I had learned that our loving Heavenly Father doesn't mind providing assurances for every one of life's challenges, regardless of their frequency or difficulty. He knows we are human. Psalm 103 says, *"He remembers that we are dust."* God doesn't expect us, as fearful, weak human beings, to experience a one-time assurance that lasts forever. So, in answer to my prayer, he gave me Psalm 91:5-6 as an assurance for my second chemotherapy treatment. It says in part:

You will not fear the pestilence that stalks in darkness, or the destruction that wasteth at noonday...

The incredible impact of this fresh assurance was from the very descriptive words found in this verse. The doctors and nurses at St. Vincent hospital had always referred to acute myeloid leukemia (AML) as a silent stalker. You have AML, but you don't know you have it. You only feel a tiredness of body and you rationalize the tiredness away. But, the silent stalker keeps stalking you until it slips up and captures you before you have any idea of how much danger you are in. Knowing all about silent stalkers, God responds with, "You will not fear the pestilence that *stalks* in darkness, or the destruction that wasteth at noonday." Or, in other words, "Tom, don't be afraid of the silent stalker (AML), or the poison (chemotherapy) that will waste you at noonday." God's assurance was affirmed when the medical staff set my appointment for a chemo pump hook up at noon! Tears came to my eyes as I realized how faithful God was in his assurance, even down to treatment preparation details!

Many new things had to be learned during the second set of treatments, including how to clean my Hickman port at home. A home healthcare nurse came to our house and showed me how to flush the port and connecting tubes to prevent any clotting. The treatment went very well, though I occasionally struggled with panic attacks. At each occurrence, the essence of Psalm 91 would always bring me around. The words, "Don't fear the silent stalker or its destruction," passed between my lips many times!

As my immune system resistance rapidly dropped, I had to go to Indianapolis for blood tests. Though I tried to be very careful, I developed an infection, or so it appeared. The first symptom was a rising temperature. Dr. Schultz had told me that if I developed a fever, I was to come to the hospital immediately and have him paged. He was particularly concerned about staph infections, because staph can be fatal within 48 hours if it invades a compromised immune system. With my immune level at 0.0, I could be in mortal peril within a very short period of time. Following the doctor's counsel, I went back to St. Vincent's hospital, paged Dr. Shultz, and ended up being readmitted. I stayed for two weeks, as the medical staff pumped me full of antibiotics to counteract the infection. Our congregation immediately initiated a prayer chain. To this day, no one knows what the actual problem was. Cultures of my blood showed no evidence of an infection even though I was in the hospital for 14 days. Though my situation was mystifying, God continued to assure me of his promises and his presence. He gave me the daily strength to endure the treatment, and sent me encouragement in various ways. My heart breaks for people who have no family, and very few friends. While I felt unworthy of, and guilty about, all of the care and concern that was showered upon me, I was so grateful for the faithfulness of God.

Shortly after being discharged from the hospital for the second time, my dear father died. I was home alone, listening to a sectional tournament basketball game, a game that the girl's team Tom coached was winning, when a phone call informed me that Dad was no longer with us. While Dad was suffering from dementia, his physical condition, especially his cardio-vascular condition, seemed pretty robust. Though I knew that he would eventually die, I wasn't expecting this "suddenness" of death. As I meditated upon his death, I had a sense, deep in my spirit, that his death, at this moment in time, had much broader and more profound meaning. For some reason, God only knows why, I sensed that my father's death was in my place. Now I know that such a conclusion may seem very unusual, or even quite strange to most people. And, perhaps they are correct, for I don't profess to understand very much about how the spiritual realm surrounding us functions. God does work in mysterious ways, his wonders to perform! What I do understand is that at the very heart of Christianity is the doctrine of substitution—the act of taking the place for someone else. Jesus stands in our place before God the Father. Substitutionary atonement means Jesus took our sins upon himself and paid our penalty for sin with his death upon the cross.

Likewise, as we embrace our Lord's example, we can "stand in the place" of others. We can make their burdens our burdens, make their sorrows our sorrows, and we can make their pain our pain. I was bowled over one day when a young Christian in our congregation told me that, after hearing I had leukemia, he prayed, "Lord, give me some of Tom's pain." Almost immediately he began feeling pain in his body. This undeniable pain remained for three weeks, and did not cease until he heard my recorded message based on the twenty-one days text found in the book of Daniel. Isn't that fascinating?

My father had "stood in" for me many times. The most recent time had been his willingness as an 80 year-old man to accept the pastorate of Skinner Worship Chapel, back when it was a congregation of 15 or 20 people, and hold it for me because he knew I would be coming back from Chicago and re-entering the pastorate. So much more could be said, and I won't labor the point, but rather affirm that I believe my father stood in my place through his death. I find it interesting that the average life expectancy of someone with acute myelogenous leukemia (AML) is ten to twelve weeks (without treatment). I was diagnosed with AML in November, and Dad died in February, ten to twelve weeks later. I would never say, in absolute terms, that these two facts are related, for I will not presume upon the mysterious ways of our loving Lord. Nevertheless, I continue to believe in my heart of hearts that Daddy died in my place.

I'm so grateful that my immune system had recovered enough so I could participate in Dad's funeral. My two brothers and I shared in the officiating responsibilities. It was a tremendous privilege to open with the song, *Thank You for Giving to the Lord,* and then spend the balance of the service celebrating Dad's life and ministry.

Following Dad's funeral, it was time for me to go back to the hospital for the final chemotherapy treatment called "High-dose Ara-C." I was somewhat concerned, as well as fearful of this treatment because it can have neurological side effects. Again, God gave me his assurance from a specific Scripture—Psalm 41:3:

> *The Lord will sustain him on his sickbed and restore him from his bed of illness.*

Sustain and restore. That was God's promise. Restore means bring back to original condition. When we restore a car, we bring it back to its original condition. Despite this high-dose Ara-C, I was going to be restored!

The final treatment went fairly well, even though I had some weakness and difficulty from its intensity. The highlight of this hospitalization was the opportunity to visit with Mrs. Lee and her husband. In a previous chapter, I told the story about Dr. Schultz coming into my room late one night and asking prayer for a woman who had been admitted with severe cancer. It was a privilege to visit with them and realize she was recovering so beautifully—a direct answer to prayer.

Following this final treatment, I returned home a happy man, even though my white cell counts were very low, and there was high potential for infection. In fact, I did experience a "scare," and had to return to the hospital for an additional two weeks. My temperature rose to 105.7°. I remember being in a kind of a semi-conscious state from the high fever, and asking God to protect my mind so that I would be able to continue to minister, study, and preach. I'm very grateful for God's sustaining and restoring touch!

I returned home pretty weak, but immediately began a consistent regimen of walking and praying. I very slowly eased my way back into a light workload at the church, and took great delight in being able to preach every Sunday. As my immune system rebuilt, I was able to be around the people in my congregation again. I was so happy to reconnect with them on a one by one basis. By June, a most beautiful month, summer was in full bloom, and my hair began to grow in again. Seeing hair on my head was restoration indeed!

I was intrigued by the fact that everywhere I went, people told me I looked ten years younger. Some even said 20 years younger. At first, I accepted their comments as a form of encouragement, until I realized they were dead serious. I was flattered by their sincerity, being 51 years old at the time, but, as the comments kept coming, tears would well up in my eyes, and I would respond, "Well, I feel younger." And, I did! Health, strength, and energy began coursing through by body in a fresh, powerful way. At my regular check-ups, Dr. Schultz was astounded at how well I was doing. Again, I thanked the Lord for his promise to sustain and restore!

As I tried to respond to people's flattering comments in a more meaningful way, including responses to the doctors and nurses at St. Vincent, I would refer to the verse God had given me through my son, Scott. From a previous chapter, you may remember the story of how Scott shared the verses in Psalm 103 with me. I was drawn to verse five:

> *He will satisfy your desires with good things, and He will renew your youth like the eagle's.*

During the previous November and December, it may have seemed surrealistic to embrace the idea that God would renew my youth. My greatest desire was to continue living and ministering. But now, only seven months later, people kept saying how much younger I seemed, and how much younger I looked. He is, indeed, the God who does abundantly more that we could ever ask, or even think!

As the summer moved along, I did a lot of reflecting on all that had happened to me. Sometimes these reflective times turned into moments of intense emotion, periods of deep emotional release. A lot had happened to me in such a short period of time, and, in some ways, I'm a "delayed reaction" kind of person. I spent hours pondering over a number of questions. Two questions in particular seemed to dominate my thinking: "Why did God choose to touch me in this manner?" and, "Why did God choose to offer me hope again and add years to my life?" I knew God is no respecter of persons. He does not choose or play favorites. So why did he grant me this unmerited favor? In the next chapter, which brings my book to an end, I will share some reasons why I believe God sustained and restored me, and added years to my life.

Chapter 11

"I've come that you might have life—
life more abundantly . . ."

"Precious is the death of His saints."

The title to this last chapter might seem contradictory, but it makes perfect sense to those who search out the meaning of the Holy Scriptures. For it was Jesus who said, "I have come that you might have life and have it more abundantly." (John 10:10) Jesus is saying that he offers his followers a fuller, deeper life, one of abundant faith, focus, and value. However, the divinely inspired Psalmist said, "Precious in the sight of the LORD is the death of his saints." (Psalm 116:15) Having gone through a near-death experience, I believe I understand, in part, what this verse means. When you are near death's door, you realize that you may actually be going to see the Lord—he who gave his life for you, he whose blood was shed for you, he who took your place on the cross. You realize that you may be seeing loved ones who have gone on before you. You realize that the heaven you've heard about, read about, and wondered about may be very near. These realizations may create a greater sense of God's presence and a more intimate closeness to him. It could well be the time when God fulfills his promise in Psalm 23:

> *Yea, though I walk through the valley of the shadow of death, I will fear no evil, for thou art with me. Thy rod and thy staff, they comfort me.*

Looking death in the face can be a very precious experience for a follower of Christ. I also believe it is a very precious experience for God. If he loves us so much that he sent his only son to die on the cross for our salvation, then we must be of great value to him. The world around us can pull us in a lot of different directions as we live our daily lives. And, there's a sense in which allowing us to live here on earth, God is taking a chance, because our choices can take us in directions away from him. On the other hand, by following in the footsteps of Jesus, we will be led in a direction toward God. Psalm 23 also says:

He leads me in the path of righteousness for his name's sake.

A righteous path ends in heaven itself. And, the scripture teaches that, when God calls us home, there will be a great reunion in heaven. No one will be more thrilled to welcome his redeemed ones to their heavenly home than God himself! Yes, God provides his children on earth with a "life more abundant," but it is nothing in comparison to the heavenly reception he has planned for his children. Their death is precious, indeed!

Why Me?

In my case, though I had looked death in the face, God had obviously delayed my call to heaven. I not only was recovering physically, but I had been stretched in amazing ways, and brought to new levels of spiritual growth and understanding. As I said in an earlier chapter, there were numerous times when I suffered feelings of guilt about being a cancer survivor. Hovering above those feelings, like a bird of prey, was the constant question, "Why me?" I began to actively seek an answer to this question.

Though I had made repeated efforts to minister to cancer patients through prayer and hospital visits, I now felt I should intentionally pursue a more formal approach to cancer patient ministry, as one way of answering this haunting question. I determined to become a volunteer hospital chaplain. Through the summer of 2006, I completed the formal training required by hospital regulations, and began returning to the sixth floor of St.

Vincent hospital one day a week. I cannot begin to describe how fulfilling it was to share the love and grace God had given me with those who were suffering what I had suffered. I was immediately accepted and embraced by almost everyone I encountered. God had given me a bridge of connection to other people—a cancer bridge. In one way or another, I could completely identify with every patient.

For example, during my hospitalizations, I had stayed in five different rooms. When I entered a patient's room wearing my chaplain's identification tag, I would introduce myself and say, "Not long ago, I was a patient here, in this very room."

"Really?" they would answer.

"Yes, I came here a year and a half ago, bleeding between my teeth and from my nose. The capillaries in my legs had burst. My white count was 137,000. I was told that I had acute myeloid leukemia."

It was a very effective way to identify with total strangers that often resulted in open hearts and receptiveness to spiritual matters. From that opening sentence, the two-way conversation began to flow. My ability to identify with the ravages of chemotherapy treatment—high temperatures, physical weakness, and emotional trauma—was a bridge to people's hearts.

Years before, I had learned that my son's drug addiction had given me a link to parents who were dealing with very troubled teenagers. People who had lost their parents would listen to me because I had experienced the deaths of my own parents. I could even identify rather quickly with a young man injured in an automobile accident and flown by helicopter to a nearby hospital, for my son, Allen, had gone through that very same experience. Now I was ministering at a new level, the level of cancer patients. And, God had given me the perfect bridge to them!

Prior to my own experience with leukemia, I had a soft spot in my heart for cancer patients. I think it developed from the desperation I had often witnessed that goes with the very idea of cancer. Many hours of my pastoral ministry had been spent at the bedsides of people dying of cancer. Now, I was dealing with far more than a soft spot. I was in hot pursuit of answering the question, "Why me?" Visiting with cancer patients took on a whole new ministry dimension. Far more was involved than my head and professional training, or a soft spot in my heart. Rather, my whole being was involved—body, soul, and spirit—in reaching out to those afflicted with this horrible disease. Now, I could identify with the patient's perspective. Every pastor needs to be a patient! And, the more I ministered to cancer patients as a former cancer patient, the more I understood God's answer to my question, "Why me?"

My volunteer, one-day per week, chaplaincy usually consisted of seeing several patients, often patients being treated by Dr. Shultz. As I walked the hospital corridors, I had to decide which patients to visit, for there were always more patients to visit than time would allow. Thus, on a warm June day, I stepped to the side of the hallway as hospital attendants pushed a patient past me wearing an oxygen mask. As I glanced to see that the patient was a moderately young woman, something spoke to me and said, "Go see that woman."

I followed the attendants to the doorway of her room and waited while they helped her get back into bed and rearrange herself. Obviously, it was not a good time for a visit, so I went off to visit other patients. Later, I came back by her room, stepped inside, introduced myself, and shared a bit of my own leukemia experience. Again, there was an immediate connection. Elizabeth was from the state of New York. While visiting a friend in Indianapolis, she experienced breathing difficulties from what she thought was congestion from an upper respiratory infection. As her conditioned worsened, she went to an emergency room, and from there was transferred to the sixth floor of St. Vincent Hospital. Specialists confirmed that she was suffering from severe lung cancer. Many miles from home and her two children, she was facing intense chemotherapy treatment all alone. It was the greatest of all privileges to offer her hope. I told her how I had survived and how God had touched me. I could quickly tell that her perilous condition had fostered a deep desire for spiritual help. I was able to secure a Bible for her and mobilized a group of prayer warriors from our church to uphold her in prayer. It wasn't long before she opened her heart to the Lord! Faced with financial difficulty, a common problem for cancer patients, our church donated over $800 for a plane ticket so Elizabeth could fly back to New York for a family visit. The radiant expression on her face said more than words could ever express!

On another occasion, I was paged by a nurse who told me of a very emotionally distraught man who had just been told that he had cancer. I went to the isolation room, put on the gown and mask, and sat with Scott, an electrician from a nearby small town. A young, strong man, Scott had never expected anything like cancer to invade his life. A husband, and father of small children, he was devastated by the grimness of his condition, wondering what would become of his family. He began to weep. My heart was moved in a way I cannot describe. As I began telling Scott about my own cancer experience, I sensed that a tremendous bridge was being built between us. And, as I prayed with Scott, I advised him that he could handle anything with the help of the Lord. Receptive to God's help, Scott opened his heart to the Lord. A year later (and I just saw Scott two weeks before writing this), he is doing quite well. There is no doubt that God has touched him.

Then there was Judy, a relative of one of our congregants. Judy was brought to the sixth floor of St. Vincent Hospital with AML, the same type of cancer that I had suffered. A lot of anxious memories were resurrected within me the day I first visited with Judy because she was bleeding between her teeth. I continued to minister to her on each visit and saw her for the last time 24 hours before she died. She, too, opened her heart to the Lord, and it was obvious that God's Spirit was dwelling within her. Judy's family asked me to conduct her funeral.

As God continued to open doors for me as a preacher, pastor, and hospital chaplain, the question, "Why me?" became less and less frequent and was replaced with thanking God for the day I was blessed with leukemia! Little did I know that there would be some additional challenges and stretching experiences in the weeks ahead.

Tested by Fire

In late August, my wife and I enthusiastically agreed to motorcycle to Tennessee over Labor Day with three couples we dearly love—Mark and Cindy Hartinger, Howard and Gail France, and Miriam and Jesse Stout. To be healthy enough to take such a trip was uplifting it itself. To spend some quality time with these couples was especially meaningful because of the roles they had played in my cancer experience. Howard is my faithful assistant pastor, Mark is a faithful accountability partner, and Miriam and Jesse are my faithful sister and brother-in-law. Our trip went well. We had a delightful time. It wasn't until we returned home that some new "stretching" began!

Prior to our trip, I had been preaching about the dangers of being attached to material things. I talked about how my cancer experience had helped me rethink my relationship to material things. "You can't take it with you" really hits home when you are hooked up to toxic chemicals that are killing all of your blood

151

cells. While I was appreciative of all of the things God had given me, I realized in a fresh new way their very limited value. To emphasize my point, I made the rather daring statement that if someone told me, while I was preaching, that my house was on fire, I wouldn't interrupt my sermon, but finish it, as long as I knew no one was in the house and no one would be hurt. Material things, including houses and lands, must never take the place of God's call upon our lives. Well, God gave me the opportunity to be tested on that statement.

With our trip almost competed, Pam and I were riding alone the last few miles having said goodbye to our dear friends. Knowing that the church youth group had planned to use our house and yard that day for one of their social get-togethers, we stopped and called Tom, our eldest son, to see if he and his family could meet us at a local Mexican restaurant in Logansport for dinner, for we didn't want to interrupt the church youth event going on at our house. After Tom agreed to meet us, we went to a Logansport park and relaxed until dinnertime. It was a very peaceful stop, jarringly interrupted by a fire engine, with lights flashing and sirens screaming, that roared past us. We didn't pay much attention to this interruption and rested quietly until it was time to ride to the restaurant.

When we arrived, Tom, who had already been seated, stood up with a very serious look on his face. He asked, "Have you talked to Kevin?"

I said, "No."

Tom said, "He's been trying to call you on your cell phone. Your house is on fire."

I couldn't believe what I was hearing! It was obvious that the recently seen fire engine had something to do with us! Pam and I immediately excused ourselves, jumped on our motorcycle, and headed for the house.

As we approached our home, we saw cars lined up and down the lane pointing to a mass of fire trucks and emergency vehicles. Driving the motorcycle slowly up the lane, we could tell that while the firemen were bringing the blaze under control, our home would be a total loss. Spotting 20 to 25 young people standing along the fence watching the house burn, I felt God speak to me and say, "Tom, I'm giving you an opportunity to model how a Christian man reacts when he loses his home." God's prompting set the tone for any reaction I might have developed to this staggering loss. Incredible as it might seem, God was providing me an opportunity to minister to several precious young people—kids from non-Christian homes who were just beginning to be impacted by Christian example—and demonstrate what trusting in the Lord really means! "How would I react?," wasn't the question. "How did God want me to react in this time of testing?," was the critical issue. Once again, I sensed that God was very close. I felt a deep sense of peace and stillness.

My biggest concern was that perhaps one of sons, Kevin or Scott, who were staying at home while we were gone, would feel that the fire was, in some way, their fault. We found out later that the fire was caused accidentally by uncontrollable circumstances. They had been outside helping the group members ride horses on the trails around our house. When they came back, one of the young women had gone into the house to use the bathroom, only to find that a glass bowl holding a scented burning candle had shattered and started a raging fire.

As I said before, the house was a total loss. I remember standing in the front yard watching the firemen trying to put out the flames that were coming from the part of the roof that hadn't already collapsed. As I watched, the fire chief said to me, "Could I ask you something?"

I said, "Sure."

He said, "Are you okay, or are you in shock?"

I said, "I'm OK, and I'm not in shock. Why do you ask?"

He said, "You're about the calmest homeowner I've ever seen at a fire."

I laughed and put my hand on his shoulder. I said, "Sir, I'm a Christian. I've followed the Lord for 34 years, and have been a minister for 24 years. I've seen a lot and have been through a lot in my life. I almost lost a son to addiction and another son to an automobile accident. My mother died in my arms a few years ago, I nearly died with leukemia a few months ago, and my father died during my chemotherapy treatments. This is just a house. No one was in it, and no one was hurt. It's okay." The fire chief grabbed me, hugged me, and said, "You know what? I've had leukemia, too!" (I found out later that he had been successfully treated for a milder form of leukemia.) It was so incredible to meet a total stranger while watching my house burn down and make such a tremendous personal connection! God is good!

That evening several friends and neighbors came by, viewed the damage and offered immediate help. We were overwhelmed with offers of personal assistance. For example, one neighbor offered us an empty parsonage owned by their church. Their pastor had accepted a call to another church and the parsonage was vacant and would remain so for some time. We ended up accepting the offer of Tom and Trisha, our son and daughter-in-law to move in with them. Even though we were down to the clothes on our backs, with everything else destroyed or damaged to the place of uselessness, Jehovah Jireh, he who goes ahead, was providing for our every need. Our problem wasn't the need for help, rather it was the problem of what help to accept!

The next morning I arose early and drove over to the house alone. I needed some time to absorb what had happened, and I was concerned for our horses. With the electrical panel destroyed, the well pump wasn't working, and there was no water supply for our thirsty animals. I remember kneeling in the grass next to the electric meter and praying, "Lord, I know you will help us get through this difficulty. I thank you for all you've done for us. I thank you for this experience. I know it's for a very good reason. You always have good reasons. But, this morning I ask you to send me some electrical help so I can water my horses." I finished the prayer, stood up, and started walking up the small rise to the burned out shell that was once our home. As I approached the house, I saw Eric Alwine driving up our lane in his truck. Eric, a dear friend, is an electrician, and does a lot of different types of contracting work. He pulled up beside me and said, "I was working on the roof of a house, and God spoke to me and said, 'Tom needs some help.' I've come to help you." Within an hour he had us hooked up to electrical power and water for our horses. God is good!

State Farm Insurance immediately sent a claims adjuster out to survey the damage. I felt some concern, for I couldn't remember the full scope of our insurance coverage. Once again, God took tremendous care of us. The way the insurance company settled with us is quite a story; the story is long, but the settlement was quick! I had asked God to give us favor with the insurance company and to guide us in all of the settlement details. State Farm showed incredible kindness to us, and Jeff Becker, our insurance adjuster, became a friend, confidant, and helper through this difficult time.

While waiting for the settlement to take place, I had an opportunity to speak at a cancer fund-raising banquet in Indianapolis. I had been asked to share the story about my cancer experience, and to offer hope to cancer patients and their families. It was affirming to see how my personal experiences ministered to others, including the current experience of recovering from a fire. Following the banquet, as I was shaking hands with various people and getting ready to leave, a woman, a total stranger, came up to me, looked me straight in the eye, and, in a kind of street lingo said, "God gonna give you double for your trouble." I kind of laughed, said thank you, and walked away. But, her statement lingered in my mind—double for your trouble! Little did I know that God was, indeed, going to give me double for my trouble. The bottom line? We were able to build a new house (same location) in the next three months that had twice the value of the house that burned. I won't describe all of the details of how the church gave me an extended leave, and with the help of many accomplished friends, we did a lot of the construction work ourselves. When the settlement was complete, we had a new home with an appraised value double that of our previous house, new furnishings for every room, a wardrobe of new clothes, and a new vehicle to drive! If that wasn't enough, my sons, who helped with the reconstruction, were amazed that I could carry 90-pound bundles of shingles up a ladder to the roof. Less than a year previously, I was too weak to walk across a hospital room. God is good!

Expanding Our Territory

As I bring this book to a close, I want to back up a little bit and share an event that happened about a month after the fire, while we were rebuilding our new home. It speaks to the question I asked at the beginning of this chapter, "Why me?" Why was I blessed in such a marvelous way by both physical healing and the restoration of my home by a God who never plays favorites?

This event started when I found a message on my cell phone voicemail, a message that was hard to understand, for the person who left the message was crying while trying to record at the same time. As I continued to listen, I realized it was the voice of

Kathy Hinds, my sister-in-law. Perhaps you remember that Kathy was the one who had given me the word from the Lord found in II Kings, verse 20, the word that said the Lord was going to heal me and add years to my life. In her broken voice, she said, "Tom, I have something I must tell you. Early this morning I was asking God, 'Why is all this difficulty happening to Tom and Pam? Now, they've had a fire!' And, God spoke very clearly to me that he was expanding your territory." She sobbed some more, and the message ended. I saved the message, and in the next few weeks, listened to it a number of times. Over and over in my mind I would hear the words "expand your territory." I had lots of time to pray as I worked with my hands on the house. Sometimes I would get up very early and go to the partially built house to think and pray before the other workers arrived. I began probing with the Lord about what "expand your territory" really meant. If my cancer and fire experience were a means of expanding our territory, what was the territory, and how was it going to expand? Was the church going to go through a burst of incredible growth? Would we be dealing with multiples of new people requiring additional services and larger facilities?

As I contemplated these questions and the possible answers to them, God began speaking to me from a passage of scripture that he had given me years before, one I referred to in an earlier chapter. It is a passage that has been a guiding light for my ministry. Luke 14:16-24 tells the story of a well to do master that prepared a magnificent banquet and invited an impressive list of guests. He was dumbfounded when they declined his invitation and offered the lamest excuses. Though the master was very unhappy about how his invitation was refused, rather than cancel the supper the master mandated his servants to invite the crippled, the lame, the halt, and the blind. After doing so, the servants came back and told him that many were coming, but there still was room for more. So the master said, "Go out to the highways and hedges—to the broken people, the wayward people, the troubled people that no one would want—and compel them come. I want them at my supper."

I trust my paraphrased way of retelling this story clearly communicates God's heart for the broken and troubled people of this world. It is the story that captures the heart of the Gospel itself—the Good News. It emphasizes what Jesus announced to the whole world in his very first sermon in Luke 4:18-19:

> *The Spirit of the Lord is on me. He has anointed me to preach good news to the poor. He has sent me to proclaim freedom and deliverance for the prisoners and to give sight to the blind, to set the captives free, to release the oppressed, to heal the broken-hearted, and to proclaim the year of the Lord's favor.*

The mission of Jesus was to reach the lost and the hurting. While I was pondering, "Expand our territory; what does that mean?," God was reminding me of the mission of Jesus through a scripture with which I was most familiar. The dots began to connect. The questions, "Why me?," "Why an extension of my life?," and "What does an expansion of my territory really mean?," seemed to be connected together by the mission of Jesus as stated in Luke, chapter four.

My thinking was illuminated even further as I was walking by the river one day, taking some time away from the construction work to think and pray. I sensed God speaking to me from the eighth chapter of Luke, especially through verses 22-56. Before I review those verses, I need to say that dominating my thoughts as I pondered these verses were two words: rescue resort. Years earlier my son Scott had gone through addiction rehabilitation in Western Michigan at the Teen Challenge rehabilitation facility. While visiting him and attending his graduation from their program, my wife and I were impressed by how "broken people" were restored to a healthy, productive life. I'll never forget some of the testimonies we heard from drug addicts at the graduation ceremony who had found a new life through their faith in Jesus Christ. During our four-hour drive home that night, we were close to tears. As we continued talking, we realized we both felt the same thing—that at some point in our lives, God wanted us to develop and create a place for the troubled, broken people in our immediate area of ministry.

As the words "rescue resort" dominated my thinking, I realized that this was the answer that connected all of my questions for the past several months. God wanted us to develop and create a place of help—"a magnificent banquet"—for troubled, broken people. He wanted a home-like place in our ministry area where people who had been abused, were addicted to drugs, or were deeply damaged by broken families, could be taken in and ministered to for protracted periods of time. This wasn't to become an institution, but a home with godly, well-trained house parents who with the assistance from the staff and laypeople of our church, would minister to, and care for the "highways and hedges" people. It was to become a rescue resort for recovery, a place where a fresh start could be found, additional education could be arranged, a job could be secured, and a life put on the track of God's blessing and help.

I realized this was a huge undertaking. To do this properly, we would need two structures, one for men and one for women. A dedicated team with exceptional counseling skills would be required, as well as people who understood and identified with these kinds of problems. Both my son and one of our assistant pastors who had recovered from drug addictions came to mind. I imagined how Scott and Mike would work one-on-one with former drug addicts and help them find a fresh start. Other people started coming to mind that had expressed an interest in helping "down and out" people.

Luke, chapter eight, describes four miracles of Jesus. As the Lord walked me slowly through this scriptural passage, I began weeping, realizing the perfect parallel it spelled out for future ministry. The four miracles are: 1) calming the storm, 2) delivering the demoniac, 3) healing the woman with blood disease, and 4) raising a young girl from the dead. God reminded me very clearly how 1987 to 1997 had been a very stormy period in my life. It was a tumultuous decade of trying to help scores of troubled people as a small church pastor, while raising a family on a meager income. It was a time when one son succumbed to a very difficult period of drug addiction and another son spent two years in rehabilitation from a near fatal automobile accident. It was a decade of the most difficult kinds of pastoral counseling problems—funerals for six year-old boys who shot themselves through the heart with a revolver, or twenty year olds killed in a bar fight. It was, indeed, a time of great stress in our marriage due to all of the difficulties and pressures. And, the word "stormy" doesn't quite capture all that filled our everyday lives and ministry. But, the first story in Luke, chapter eight, tells how Jesus calmed the Sea of Galilee storm by rebuking it, as well as his disciples for their lack of faith, and reports that the storm was followed by a great calm.

Following the calm, and the crossing of the Sea of Galilee, the second story tells how Jesus was approached by a man possessed by a thousand demons, a man who screamed while scraping himself with stones in attempts at self destruction. Jesus addressed him, rebuked the demons, and the scripture says the man accepted clothes and fellowshipped with Jesus and his disciples "in his right mind."

God showed me that this was the second segment of our ministry, the period of time when we were called to minister on the streets of Chicago. As I have described, we had to double our prayer time in order to deal with the evil forces that were working those streets, especially in the darkness of night. We actually encountered troubled people who would literally jump up and down and scream at us as we attempted to minister to them. It was a time of dealing with the evil one on a face-to-face level. This spiritual warfare hit home when our son, who had been in the automobile accident, attempted suicide by slashing himself with a knife. He was almost successful. I sensed, at the time, that this action was a definite attempt on the part of the evil one to destroy and kill him. And, it was during this time in Chicago that my nerves fell apart, and I had a complete nervous breakdown, while watching the church I was trying to establish begin to be ripped apart. I had to take six months off to get back to my senses. Like this second story in Luke, chapter eight, Jesus rebuked the powers of darkness, and restored this very distressed person to health and wholeness, and then advised him to "return home." At the end of our Chicago experience of dealing with the demonic, we returned home. God led us back to central Indiana and a Skinner Chapel pastorate.

The third story is about the woman with a blood disease. It begins as Jesus responds to the plea of Jairus to come and heal his very sick daughter. The scripture says that as Jesus was walking along, a growing crowd of people joined in the walk with him. I was immediately able to relate to this story, for within months of accepting a call to Skinner Chapel, it was necessary to build an additional building to house the growing number of people who wanted to "walk" with us, and develop an effective outreach ministry in our area. But, as Jesus walked, there was an interruption of his journey by a woman who had suffered some kind of blood disease for many years. Oh, how clearly God reminded me that, as God had blessed, the crowd had come, and the ministry had flourished. We were on our way, rescuing and helping people. Then, there was a huge interruption—a blood disease that nearly took my life. Through

161

the power of simply touching the hem of Jesus' garment, the woman was healed. In the same way, as people had prayed for me—people who reached out and touched God on my behalf—I, too, was healed. The Luke story goes on to say that she came trembling, and bowed and thanked Jesus for the tremendous miracle he had performed. I paused in my reading of this story, overwhelmed with gratitude for what the Lord had done for me!

Jesus finally arrived at the home of Jairus only to be told that the little girl had died. Unfazed by this news, Jesus asked Peter, James, John, and her parents to join him as he took the dead girl's hand and said, "My child, get up!" In a very personal way, Jesus took her by the hand and gave life back to her. I continued to weep as I realized God was showing me that, by his grace and goodness, we had survived the stormy decade of 1987 to 1997, and our intense and brutal encounter with the demonic in Chicago. Now after experiencing an almost fatal blood disease, I was to offer life back to young people, people whose lives were being destroyed by various forms of abuse. We were to offer life to those "dead" in their trespasses and sin, and give them new life in Jesus Christ.

God had answered the question, "Why me?" It all made perfect sense. Luke, chapter eight, was a full confirmation of the Rescue Resort concept I had been thinking about for some time. God wanted us, in a very personal way, to provide a spiritual, emotional, and physical home for those trapped and lost in the highways and hedges of this world. God wanted us to take "the least of these" by the hand and offer them "the way, the truth, and the life."

So, here we are. As I pen these words, we are working on opening the women's section of the Rescue Resort in the near future. Eventually, we hope to purchase a large parcel of land, where we intend to put up two structures (one home for young men, one home for young women) on each end of the property.

This will be a place where the hurting and the broken can come for three months, six months, or a year to be nursed back to life by house parents and other caring people—a minister, a chaplain, a counselor, a doctor.

How reassuring it is to have an answer to the question "Why me?"

The bridge I have to cancer patients, I intend to transverse the rest of my life. Even this past week, I visited a number of patients, offering them hope and salvation, and praying for their healing, as God wills. We must respond to the directive of our Master and take every opportunity to fill his banquet table with those who are hurting, down and out, and broken. Nothing pleases him more. What an awesome privilege to help "bring them in" from the highways and hedges. What an awesome responsibility! May God help us to be faithful to his call.

May God be praised!

Thank You

Two weeks after finishing the manuscript for this book, a wonderful lady I had gotten acquainted with, Margaret Cook, died with AML. Five days before dying, she opened her heart to the Lord and asked me to have her funeral. I had her funeral and met her three wonderful adult children. The first money given for publication of this book came from Margaret. How special.

I want to especially thank Rae Bates for her work on preparing this book. I could not have done it alone. She and her husband, Chris, have been a great help and encouragement in our ministry.

Thank you to all who read through the rough drafts of this book. Your input and help were instrumental in helping to make it accurate and readable. A special thanks to Paul and Mary Robbins for lending his expertise and her skills to the process.

Thank you to Sarah Reese for the cover photo.

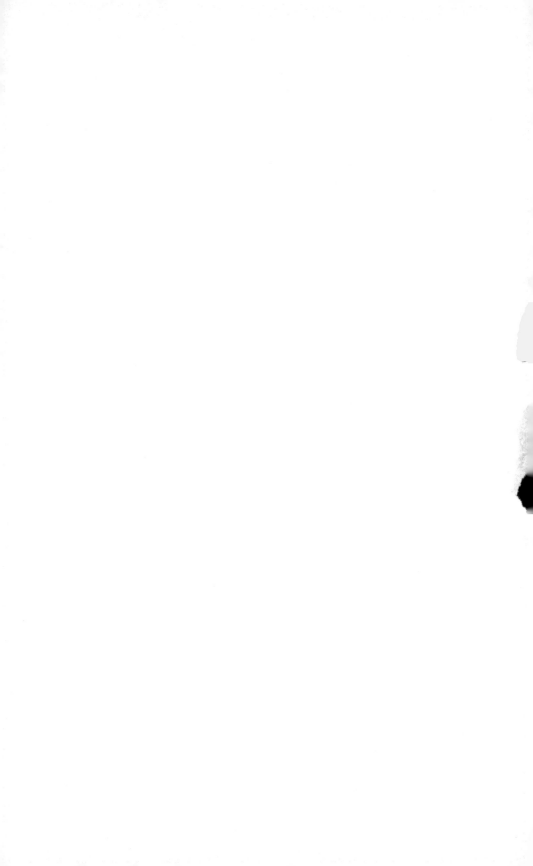

Made in the USA
Middletown, DE
06 July 2022